TURNING BOYS INTO MEN II
A MULTICULTURAL
BEHAVIORAL APPROACH

YOUTH WORKBOOK

LESSONS 1-15 COMBINED

BY DR. JAMES PARKER GRIFFIN, JR.

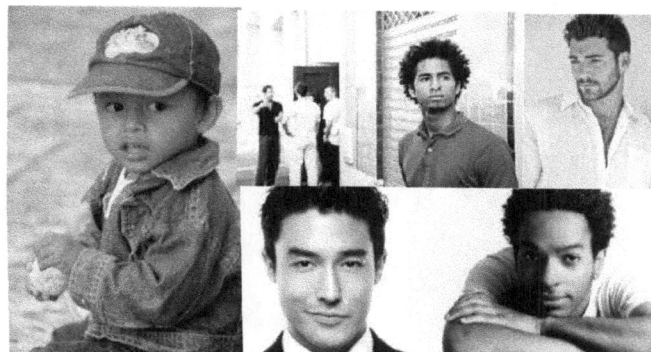

TURNING BOYS INTO MEN II

A MULTICULTURAL BEHAVIORAL APPROACH

LESSON TOPICS

1. INTRODUCTION TO MANHOOD

2. PREPARING BOYS TO BE MEN WHO LEAD

3. SUPPORTING YOUR PEERS

4. HEALTH AND FITNESS

5. MALE- FEMALE RELATIONSHIPS

6. RESPECT FOR WOMEN--PART 1

7. RESPECT FOR WOMEN--PART 2

8. FATHERHOOD

9. MANHOOD AND MASS MEDIA:
    SENSE OF MUSIC, TELEVISION, AND PRINT

10. HOW TO HANDLE PEOPLE WHO TREAT YOU UNFAIRLY

11. HOW TO DEAL WITH AUTHORITIES

12. LEARNING TO PREVENT VIOLENCE, MANAGE CONFLICT,
    AND SELECT REAL FRIENDS

13. SPIRITUALITY

14. FAST MONEY VS. HONEST MONEY: BECOMING A
    SUCCESS

15. BECOMING A MATURE, WELL-ROUNDED MAN

WHAT IS THE PURPOSE OF THE

MANHOOD DEVELOPMENT GUIDE?

This guide is designed to help young males to increase awareness and gain skills to develop into mature men in their personal, family, and community relationships. The activities in this guide will help you to acquire:

- Leadership skills
- Relationship building skills
  -Brother to brother
  -Male to female
- A clear idea of who you are
- Promote responsible self-love
- New ways of thinking
- Ways to stay out of trouble
- Accelerated pathways to success
- Taking responsibility in family and community
- Promote consideration for other people

To obtain the maximum benefits of this guide, it is important for you to remain actively involved during each exercise. The guide will help you discover success if you use it.

An important aim of this program is to encourage teenage and young adult males to become leaders. This can take place on different levels. These include acting like a boy with no leadership qualities, or not showing Leadership skills on the individual, boss, community, or National level. This training focuses on helping you move to the adult level of leadership let's look at what these levels can look like.

LEADERSHIP TYPE& AN EXAMPLE OF A PERSON(S) IN EACH GROUP	IMPORTANTACTIONSBY LEADERSHIP LEVEL
COMPLETE COUNTRIES OR THE WHOLE WOR.LD LEADERSHIP **IV** THE PRESIDENT	CHAMPIONS A CAUSE, PROMOTES A BENEFICIAL MISSION FOROTHERS IN SOCIETY.
COMMUNITY AND ORGANIZATIONS Group LEADERSH IP **III.** CHIEF EXECUTIVE OFFICER FOR A COMPANY OR SMALL BUSINESS OWNER,. FAITH LEADERSHIP FOR A CONGREGATION ETC.	SUPERVISES PEOPLE MANAGES PROJECTS ADM INI STERS PROGRAS RUNS COMPANIES OR ORGANIZATION S
MEN INDIVIDUAL LEADERSHIP **II.** MOST WORK SUPPORT	WORKING TOWARD STANDARDS. GROOMING ONESELF TO BECOME RESPONSIBLE MANAVOIDING PROCRASTINATION AND NEGATIVITY. THINKS FOR HIMSELF AND OTHERS COMMITTED TO PROMOTINGBENEFICIAL CONDITIONS FORCHILDREN, FRIENDS, FAMILY, AND THE COMMUNITY.
BOYHOOD **I.**	LACKING IN RESPONSIBLE ACTIONS REGARDING HIMSELF AND OTHERS; UNAWARE OF WAYS TO BEH AVE LIKE A MATURE PERSON; DEPENDS ON OTHERS INSTEAD OF HIMSELF.

TURNING BOYS INTO MEN II
A MULTICULTURAL BEHAVIORAL APPROACH

LESSON 1
Introduction to Manhood Development

Learning Objectives

You should learn:

- ❖ What characteristics define manhood?
- ❖ What cultural points of view help shape your personal values regarding manhood?
- ❖ What behaviors distinguish men from boys?

EXERCISE 1.1

What is MANHOOD?

STEPS: What you do

Take 5 minutes to think about the ways that you see what the word manhood means to you.

MANHOOD QUALITIES	
LIST 5 THINGS THAT SHOW THE DIFFERENCE BETWEEN A BOY AND A MAN.	
1. A boy is	a man is
2. A boy is	a man is
3. A boy is	a man is
4. A boy is	a man is
5. A boy is	a man is

EXERCISE 1.2

MEN: MOVING TOWARD SUCCESS
BOYHOOD TO MANHOOD

FUTURE MALE LEADER
YOUR ROAD TO SUCCESS

An important part of the way a mature male act is that he plans his life in a direction that moves toward being financially responsible he recognizes that if he does not look out for his success, there is no guarantee that anyone else will. This involves taking an active role in mastering the skills that lead to success. He avoids thinking negatively about other. people (from other countries for example) who make great sacrifices in order to become successful themselves instead, the mature man tries to learn from the successes of other people around him, he imitates success and combines imitation with high motivation in order to excel instead of complaining about the great opportunities that others have, he searches for or creates his own opportunities he recognizes that part of success is a series of short-term setbacks. Therefore, he never gives up on a goal and looks for ways to rise above setbacks when they occur. He views these setbacks as temporary obstacles that he will overcome eventually if he never stops trying.

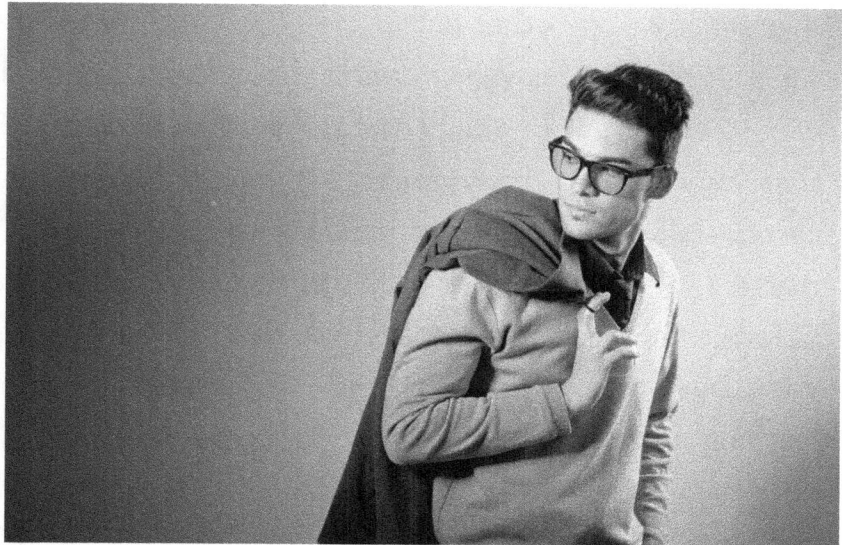

The mature guy looks at people and situations around him and anticipates which opportunities exist for self-improvement and for increasing his wealth and his health this includes working hard to become as healthy as he can, both physically and mentally more information on this subject appears in some of the later lessons in the training.

Of course, money is not everything when it comes to being a successful mature leaders understand that there are more important things in life than money alone. Some of them include developing self- respect, respect for others, integrity, character and decency taking the initiative to cultivate these qualities within you is an important part of being a whole man. The key to planning your life is to become a self-starter and to create balance in your life so that no single part of your life overshadows any other part.

Although it is very important to work to generate income, it is not the only way to express your ability as a self-starter, being a self- starter is an important skill that cuts across many areas for example, the mature male leader must be responsible for actively organizing and maintaining his living quarters, family matters, and work responsibilities to name a few. In the future, more than ever before, men who are leaders will need to be self-starters to compete in world-wide businesses that are developing across the globe motivating yourself and learning how to get along with people different from you will be absolutely necessary to achieve success in the future regardless of a person's race, ethnic background, or religious beliefs.

EXERCISE 1.3

RESPONSIBLE MEN: DEFINING WHAT THEY DO STEPS: WHAT YOU DO

STUDY THE FOLLOWING DEFINITION; WHAT IS A MATURE MALE?
WORKING DEFINITION: MATURE MALE

As early as twelve years old, a truly mature male act responsibly towards his friends, family, community, women, and children by acting in ways to please them. Males who hit women or take advantage of them sexually are not real men. Real men only teardown parts of the community when it is necessary to build something new, like a shopping center or housing development. Real men work to make people, places, and things better than they were when they first came into contact with them. This is what tells you that a guy is a mature man and a true leader

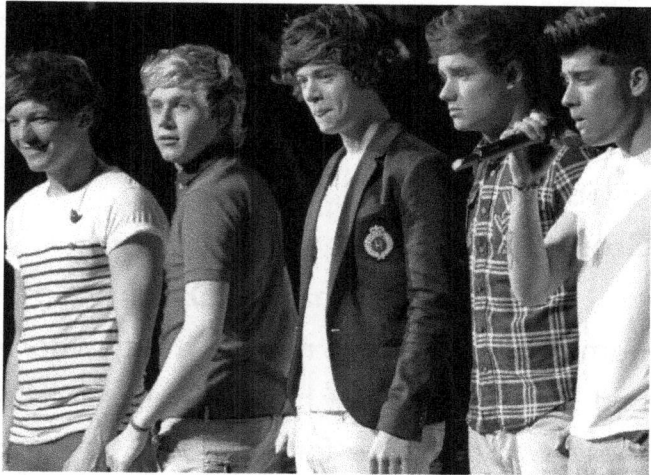

STEPS: WHAT YOU DO

Read the stories on the next page then go through the mature or less mature table (I) to identify the matching manhood traits.

Story A

Tony is a 21-year-old man who lives on the southeast side of a large urban city. He has been dating Andrea for three years. They have had talks about getting married, but there are problems that some problems stem from some of Tony's actions. Andrea recently went to the department store in order to purchase some new shoes. She discovered that her $8,000 credit card limit had been maxed. This incident occurred a week after learning that Tony had made $700 worth of long-distance telephone calls on her home phone. Tony has been using Andrea's car and returning it with the gas needle on empty. Once he offered to make up for running the gas out of the car by giving her a $5.00 bill. When Andrea demanded that Tony pays for his bills, he slapped her, knocking her to the ground. He then laughed at her and said, "You fool. I'm a man, and I do what I want to do when I get ready to do it. If you don't like it, you can find some other chump to hang out with." Andrea said, "How dare you?" Tony slapped her again and said, "How dare I what?" Andrea ran into the bathroom, locked the door behind her, and called the police. Tony was arrested; he, spent two weeks and lost his job.

Use Table 1 to identify characteristics in Column A or Column B that describe

Write them here:
Story B

A young man named David was riding the five o'clock subway on his way home from work. He noticed a lady who appeared to be about 65 years-old board and standing front of him. She appeared to be dead tired. The train was full and there was nowhere for her to sit. In an act of kindness and consideration, David gave the older lady his seat. Just then his friends started to act inappropriately, talking loudly and cursing without any consideration for anyone around them. David asked his friends to stop cursing as matter of respect for the older lady. One of his friends said, "Man you don't ever want to have any fun: · at the same time, the friends complied with David's request. Looking at the older lady, some nodded and one said he was sorry for their behavior. The lady expressed her sincere appreciation to them and smiled. David told the older lady "A real man doesn't have to curse in order to get his point across. I'm sorry, ma'am, that we didn't show more respect for you or ourselves:'
Use Table 1 to identify traits in Column A or Column B that describe.

10

Story C

Michael Payne consistently takes care of his two children, ages 2 and 4, while his girlfriend often goes to nightclubs with her friends. Michael takes his children to the park to spend time with them, and to stores to buy them clothes. He enjoys laughing with them and giving them hugs and kisses. His friends see him as a softy. Some told him that it was not his job to be "taking care of the kids." "Let their mama do that stuff," they insisted. They even went so far as to tell Michael that he should not just have one woman. "Date as many women as you can," they said. Michael told his friends they were wrong and to "mind their own business." Instead of being persuaded, Michael began to back away from his buddies from high school. He made a point to see them less and less.

Story D

Two brothers were running late to board a plane. It would have taken two hours to drive to the airport and park, so they decided to take the rail system. As they walked toward the rail system, three guys with guns stopped them. It was dark outside, and no one else was near. The situation caught them off guard. The three-armed men surrounded them. One of the brothers said, "Whatever you guys want, you can have. We don't have any cash." Two of the men began to reach for the brothers' luggage. When they did this, the brothers started yelling for help and began to run in front of the approaching cars. One of the cars happened to be a police car. The policeman drove onto the sidewalk between the brothers. The officers had now drawn their guns and one shouted, "Drop your weapons!" When one of the robbers refused to drop his weapon, one of the officers shot two of the criminals. One of the men died at the scene and the other two were taken into custody.

Use Table 1 to identify characteristics in Column A or Column B that describe the brothers and the robbers.

WAYS TO DESCRIBE MATURE AND LESS MATURE

TABLE 1: MANHOOD DEVELOPMENT

COLUMN A; MEN	COLUMN B; BOYS
1.Demonstrate responsibility for his actions	1.Remains self-centered
2.Consider other people feelings routinely	2.Easily influenced by peers
3. Promote non-violence with people who lived around him.	3.Ruins people and places around him
4.Earns items that he uses personally	4. React to negative events rather than avoiding them.
5.Respect people	5.Physically mistreat women
6.Respect property	6. Think of self-more often than others.
7.Obeys the law	7. Accepts twisted ideas without considering their effect on others.
8.Promote people healthy thoughts	8.Starts conflicts
9.Shows self-control	9.Uses belongings of others without permission
10.Maintains self-discipline	10.Takes advantages of women's belonging
11.Make people around him stronger	11.Share little of himself with the community
12.Displays patience	12.Insist that self-restraint is pointless
13.Complete tasks without quitting	13.Jump from one project to another prematurely
14.Tolerate others	14.Get Drunk or high when he feels like it
15.Gives back to the community	
16. Keeps his body away from toxic substances like alcohol and drugs.	

TURNING BOYS INTO MEN II
PREPARING BOYS
TO BE MEN WHO LEAD

LESSON 2

LEARNING OBJECTIVE

YOU SHOULD LEARN;
    1. WHAT BEHAVIORS DISTINGUISH MEN FROM BOYS?

EXERCISE 2.1
MANHOOD LEADERSHIP: RAP-PLEDGE WRITING EXERCISE
STEPS: WHAT YOU DO

Take 10 minutes to write a personal rap or Pledge About becoming a male leader... Describe the ideal way you would like to see yourself 25 years from now. You can refer to Exercise 1.3 for the definition of a mature male leader. To see what characteristics, you want to adopt.

EXAMPLE OF A MANHOOD RAP FROM A YOUNG GUY	WRITE YOUR OWN RAP, POEM, OR STATEMENT BELOW DESCRIBING THE WAY THE IDEAL MAN BEHAVES.
To define being a man, you must follow these steps. The truth is hard, so is the pill you must swallow.	
Patience is the key to big success. Having self-discipline gets rid of the stress.	
A grown man accepts others and obeys the law. He respects himself and boosts healthy thoughts.	
He's responsible for. His own actions. Earning his way gives him satisfaction.	
Never Does he give up or Promote violence. He also understands the concept of guidance.	
He knows the value of hugs and What drugs do to you? No, he's not Self-centered nor. Influenced by cruel peers. He treats girls right. He's becoming a grown man tonight.	

TURNING BOYS INTO MEN II PREPARING BOYS TO BE MEN WHO LEAD
LESSON 2

One of the most important ways to be a respectable man is to have standards, values, and ideals that place limits on what actions are acceptable and what behaviors are unsatisfactory.

Different cultures have various standards for the way that mature men behave. The key to being an emotionally and physically healthy man is to embrace a set of standards to uphold. Here are some examples. Which ones work best for you?

EXERCISE 2.2

MANHOOD DEVELOPMENT CODES OF CONDUCT: DISCUSSION. CHECK OUT THESE MANHOOD STANDARDS AND SEE WHICH ONES WORK BEST FOR YOU EXPLAIN WHY THESE GUIDELINES FOR BEING A MATURE MAN FIT YOUR SITUATION.

AMERICAN BOY SCOUT LAW

A scout is:

- Trustworthy
- Loyal
- Helpful
- Friendly
- Courteous
- Kind
- Obedient
- Cheerful
- Thrift
- Brave
- Clean
- Reverent

How well does the Boy Scout code fit the lifestyle of young people today? How would you change it to fit today's youth or are these standards timeless? Explain why.

NGUZA SABA PRINCIPLES
BY DR. MAULANA KARENGA

1. **Unity (Umoja):** To strive for and maintain unity in the family, community, nation, and race.

2. **Self-Determination (Kujichijulia):** To define ourselves, Name ourselves, and speak for yourselves instead of being defined and spoken for by others.

3. **Collective Work and Responsibility (Ujima):** To build and maintain our Community together; to make our brothers' and sisters' problems our problems, and to solve these problems together.

4. **Cooperative Economics (Ujamaa):** To build and own stores, shops, and other businesses, and profit together from them.

5. **Purpose (Nia):** To make as our collective vocation the building and development of our community in order to restore people to their_ traditional greatness.

6. **Creativity (Kuumba):** To always do as much as we can, in the way we can, so as to leave our community more beautiful and beneficial than when we inherited it.

7. **Faith (Imani):** To believe, regardless of what others say, in our parents, our teachers, our leaders, our people, and us, and the righteousness and victory of our struggle.

EXERCISE 2.3 (CONTINUED)

HERE IS ANOTHER CODE OF CONDUCT WHICH DAVID HEISMAN CREATED.
HIS CODE OF CONDUCT CONSISTS OF THE FOLLOWING STANDARDS:

1. I am a man of the 21st century I live true to my values and principles and chase my goals even if it means my own death.

2. I am an entrepreneur, I choose to calculate risks and act decisively, and I choose to make Mistakes of ambition over mistakes of sloth.

3. I choose to mar.ch to my own tune and my tune alone I choose to help others not out of obligation but out of compassion, love, and respect.

4. I remember that fortune is a wave with peaks and troughs I celebrate and enjoy the highs, and I'm grateful and resilient during the lows.

5. My life has value. It is up to me and me alone to prove this value to the world. No one else is going to fight for my economic freedom but me and me alone.

6. I choose to view each new day as a new page in the story of my life. I am free to fill that page how I like, regardless of what has happened in the past.

7. I understand that there is no excuse or rationalization that is stopping me from getting what I want but that of my own fear. I choose to look at this fear to accept this fear and to take action because action cures fear.

8. Finally, I view life as my persona playground. Play helps to access creativity. Creativity is the very essence of divinity.

EXERCISE 2.2 (CONTINUED)

PERSONAL CODE OF CONDUCT OF MATT GOLDENBERG

Matt Goldenberg is the founder of self-m ad e renegade, a career co ach in g firm that helps college grads and career changers get hired without the right degree, connections, or work experience.

I am the genesis of a hero, a creator, a monk, and a child. I aim to journey on, create, experience e, and play with life. My core is not limited by or defined by these personality traits, rather, it limits and defines them. These traits are both prescriptive of what I can and should at my best, and descriptive of what I cannot help even at my worst. Life is my journey, my sanctuary, my playground, my bedroom, and above all, my creation. I am a hero. I fight for who I am and what I believe. I recognize that Life is fleeting, and can end in an instant, so consciously work to make sure I am achieving life with ever y breath. I know that I must work, fight and suffer along this road; that I must do what needs to be done to learn the lessons I need, to struggle and return victorious. As the hero, I seek to follow my purpose and defeat the challenges along the way. I recognize that while death is to be fought and avoided at all costs, a life without purpose is a fate worse than death.

I am a monk, I immerse myself in the experience of life in this moment. I appreciate the majesty of life as an end in itself. I hold my focus as my greatest gift, and consciously direct it to experience life. I recognize that while planning for the future and learn in g from the past are important, I must be willing to die at any moment, and if I die, I must die fully immersed in the present. I have an affinity with nature and with other humans, as when I am immersed in the moment, I can empathize with the rhythms of nature and the feelings of others. At all times, my deepest core is at pea c e, even in the presence of great outside stressors.

I am a creator, I create the world around me and within me as I see fit. I use my unlimited power and will to change the future. My will is my greatest tool with which I can create and change the world. My work ethic is unparalleled, and this is what allows me to create such great works. I create things out of passion, out of joy, out of expression; things that are astounding, that express who I am, and enhance others' lives. As a creator, I know my body may die, but I will not, as I will live on in my creations, which are and always will be created in my image. I radiate a force and power tangible to all who come in contact with me. I am a man who moves the world.

I am a child, I seek to immerse myself in joy and love free of self-consciousness or pretension. I play and laugh freely, drawing those around me into a state of playfulness. My imagination is endless and wonderful, my greatest tool with which to play with the world. I can direct my innocence and imagination to solve problems in a creative fashion and see simple solution s that eludes others. I do not use play as a means to an end; it is an end in itself. Laughter is my greatest gift to the world, and happiness is my greatest gift to myself. If I must die, I will die with laughter in my heart.

EXERCISE 2.2 (CONTINUED)

How do these codes of conduct compare with each other_?

Which of these codes of conduct best fit the way that you are raised?

Which elements of these codes of conduct are most likely to help you become a well-rounded, sophisticated, considerate man?

Why should every mature man follow a code of conduct?

What do you think about the statement that every man should follow a universal code of conduct?

How well do the following universal standards of behavior work for you?

❖ Treat all people with love, acceptance, and fairness.
❖ Treat people the way that you want to be treated.

How would your Life be if everyone in the world followed this universal code of behavior?

EXERCISE 2.3
TYPES OF LOVE: SELF-ACCEPTANCE AND SELF-LOVE
BOYHOOD TO MANHOOD

LOVING YOURSELF

Self-love is one of the most important types of love that a person can have. This form of love is important because it is difficult, if not impossible, to care for other_ people in a loving way without loving yourself. Loving this way begins with acceptance.

One of the wisest things that you can do is to recognize that you are always going to be faced with the physical person that you are, unless you get surgically altered. Therefore, you should accept the person that you are

And build your manhood on that acceptance. You must be your own best friend in order to be a leader and a fully developed man. No circumstance, no condition, no loss in your life is worth sacrificing yours. You have an obligation as a man and leader to become all that you can as a person. Any self-destructive action on your part is contrary to being a mature man and a real leader.

EXERCISE 2.4
CULTIVATING BROTHERLY LOVE: SKIT COMPETITION
STEPS: WHAT YOU DO
❖ Groups of participants will create a Ujima skit on brotherly love
❖ The facilitator will rate the quality of the skits
❖ You will have 15 minutes to create ask it that uses the Ujima Principle

❖ Read the problem situation and then act out an appropriate solution to the problem

Ujima problem situation (solving your Brothers' and sisters' Problems together)

You are walking home after school. You see one of you. Best friends in an argument with his girlfriend. At first, they are staring at each other with angry facial expressions. Then they start yelling at each other, and then all of a sudden, your Best friend pushes the girl to the ground in you Skit, act out a peaceful way to keep this situation from getting any worse. Show how you could safely help your Friend and the girl resolve this impasse and work toward a better understanding for all parties involved.

EXERCISE 2.5
DEMONSTRATING CONCERN FOR OTHERS
STEPS: WHAT YOU DO
1. Groups of participants will create an Umoja skit showing concern for others
2. The facilitator will rate the quality of the skits
3. You will have 1/5 minutes to create a skit that uses the Umoja Principle
4. Read the problem situation and then act out an appropriate solution to the problem.

Umoja problem situation (maintain unity in family, community, Nation, and race)

A teenager And his 10 year old boy neighbor Are shooting hoops at the basketball court, when it's time for them to go home, the teary-eyed boy says that he doesn't want to go home because his step father is there. He is afraid to face his stepfather because the boy broke the stereo which he had been told not to touch. Develop ask it that shows the conversation between the teenager. And the boy how could you, as the teenager. In this situation show your concern in a positive manner. While depicting compassion and understanding for the boy and his stepfather?

TURNING BOYS INTO MEN
A MULTICULTURAL
BEHAVIORAL APPROACH

SUPPORTING YOUR PEERS

LESSON 3

TURNING BOYS INTO MEN II
A MULTICULTURAL BEHAVIORAL APPROACH
SUPPORTING YOUR PEERS
LESSON 3

LEARNING OBJECTIVES

YOU WILL LEARN:

❖ WAYS TO SUPPORT YOUR PEERS

❖ THE MEANING OF THE TERLLM RESILIENCY NETWORKI/NGC

EXERCISE 3.1

MUTUAL SUPPORT: FOR YOUR PEERS
STEPS: WHAT YOU DO

Read the passage below. Ask yourself, "Do I have a responsibility to help my friends and others achieve their goals and dreams?"

BOYHOOD TO MANHOOD

FOUNDATION

Boys and men

Learning to support each other

A set of skills that a young man can learn is how to support and provide genuine recognition and care for other males in their age group. The teen years are a time when many youths experiment with new roles and ways of thinking. At the same time, many seek the approval and respect of others in their age group. Youth aggressively search for friendly relationships that fulfill their need for acceptance and belonging.

At the same time, once they earn membership in a circle of friends, they feel safe enough to engage in playful teasing. In some neighborhoods, the exchange can become a source of entertainment for many of the young men. Because of the pleasure they receive from their interaction with each other, sometimes the teasing and criticism goes overboard. Part of this playfulness involves the exchange of what some would consider being insults. At other times, the insults amount to bullying. Sometimes the insults are straightforward and designed to entertain. At other times, the insults are uncomplimentary comments that turn vicious. In all cases, a mature person who is striving to be a respectable young man avoids mistreating other guys in his age group.

In the 1960s and 1970s, some young men called a similar way of exchanging insulting remarks with each other "Joning,", "playing the dozens,", or "scoring.". Some called it "clowning" ." in the Midwestand south, it was a different way of forming friendships, but there are strong similarities to the verbal exchanges that sometimes occur among some guys today. This social process concentrates on being quick-witted. The cleverer the young man is at making fun of his peers, the more entertaining are his comments to the audience of friends and peers. In this way, he gains attention, respect, and dominance over his peers.

On one level, this entertaining but aggressive style of relating to each other appears to be innocent in comparison to the more vicious style of this communication pattern. Some young men find the experience so entertaining and appealing that they taunt and tease each other on a continual basis continually. They see the exchange as being harmless. On a deeper level, the young men in this situation are able to achieve closeness and bonding through this teasing process.

Many adolescents say there is nothing bad about participating in the lighthearted teasing. However, when a male becomes 25 or 30thirty, the form of building relationships can grow into a lack of respect for or a distrust of other males. The results can become so serious that some young men become isolated from each other others become unduly suspicious of the motives of a new male acquaintance.

This mental grooming process does not occur by itself one argument is that the negative portrayal of some males on television and in movies contributes to the lack of trust, suspicion, and separation from each other failure to learn to work together can place males who are affected by it at a disadvantage in their quest to become complete, mature men.

The real question to consider is not whether teasing and insulting your male peers, who are usually your friends, is good or bad. Instead, the real question is whether there is a better and more mature way of relating to each other. In other words, could you be wasting the time and energy involved in negativity like cursing each other? Could you channel the time toward building brotherhood and encouraging other young males to achieve their goals and dreams together? Could you use this energy to build strong families, businesses, and communities?

The decision to promote each other's' success is a learned skill, and it is one that does not come naturally. Some say that often, people in society encourage negative events and negative views of events. That could include encouraging fighting and cursing at each other in movies, television, etc., as if they are acceptable roles to follow regardless of whether this is true, the situation does not have to be this way for everyone. It is possible for males to reprogram themselves through self-examination and self-study. Learning effective ways to support other young males is a skill that every truly maturing male has a responsibility to acquire.

HOW CAN I HELP A FRIEND WHO IS IN NEED? THINK OF THE FOLLOWING SITUATIONS AND FILL IN THE SPACES POSITIOVE ACTIONS YOU CAN TAKE
If my friend's family doesn't have enough food, I can help by:
If my classmate is sick, I can help by:
If my friend is lonely, I can help by:
If the boys in my community are skipping school, I can help by:
If my classmate is sad, I can help by:

EXERCISE 3.2
THE BROTHERHOOD: SPEAK.OUT GAME
STEPS: WHAT YOU DO

❖ You will break into small groups to brainstorm a list of 5 positive statements young African American males can make about each other.

❖ Select a group spokesman who will speak your group's positive statements.

❖ Each group takes turns until either time or the list runs out.

SPEAKOUT GAME STATEMENTS:
LIST 5 POSITIVE STATEMENTS TO DESCRIBE YOUR PEERS.

1.

2.

3.

4.

5.

EXERCISE 3.3
RESILIENCY: THE MALE RELATIONSHIP NETWORK
STEPS: WHAT YOU DO IN THIS EXERCISE

Consider the following definition.

What is resiliency networking?

Working definition

A male resiliency network involves forming positive, healthy relationships with males in your own age group, males older than you, and males younger than you. It involves reaching forward, side to side, and behind you to for-m a strong blanket of security, prosperity, and health. This responsibility also involves giving backing to people younger than you, helping to strengthen the community, and showing concern for the future of all people.

EXERCISE 3.4
GIVING BACK: FOR.MING THE RESILIENCY NETWORK
BOYHOOD TO MANHOOD
FOUNDATION

Giving back results in personal satisfaction learning the skill of giving back is a responsibility that males have to themselves, one another, their community, and the institutions that serve them. Mature men recognize that giving back is a way to obtain personal satisfaction and a way to add a sense of meaning to their lives. Giving back is a serious responsibility that every male must assume in order to help pr-event the harmful effects of negative influences like HIV and hepatitis infection, and violence in society today.

MANHOOD REQUIREMENT

Give back to two young people and require them to do the same with two younger than them in this way two manhood trainees become four, four become eight, and eight become 16.... the number increases in this way to build thousands and perhaps millions of positive and healthy relationships.

EXERCISE 3.5
BUILDING A RESILIENCY NETWORK
STEPS: WHAT YOU DO STUDY THE FOLLOWING DEFINITION:

Integrity: the demonstration of trustworthiness, uprightness, and dedication to doing what is right regardless of pressures to do what is wrong.

Character: the display of high regard for standards of behavior, without the need for monitoring from others;

Moral self-control and discipline; the ability to keep a good reputation by following social rules, laws, and guidelines for, the benefit of all people.

Decency: the expression of high morals and principles for living your, life; exhibiting proper, actions toward others according to a standard of courtesy for, living with respect for, other, people.

EXERCISE 3.6
COMPLAINING ABOUT OTHERS VERSUS TAKING CHARGE
BOYHOOD TO MANHOOD
FOUNDATION
PASSAGE CHOOSE A CLEAR VISION
SETTING GOALS, GOAL GETTING

Too many young males may want to place the responsibility for, their, achievement on someone else. It is a sign of immaturity. the full and final responsibility for, your, success lies with you. every person on this planet has a burden of some kind to bear older, people have to overcome battle with age

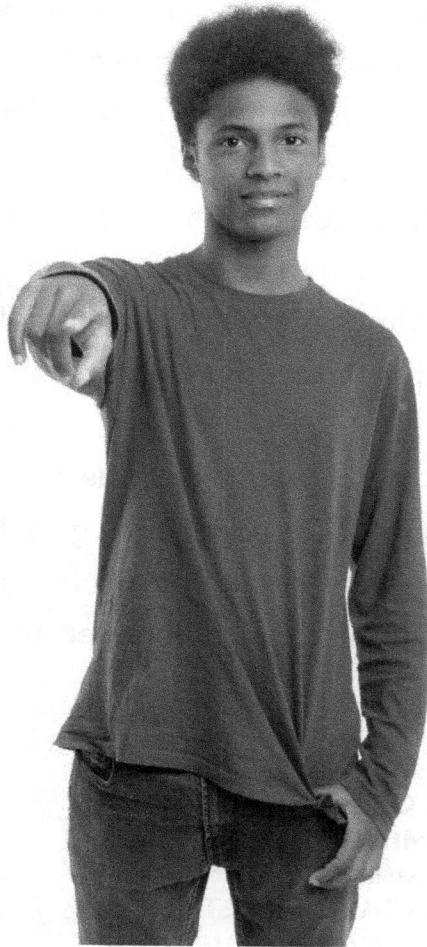

overweight people, face the challenge of dealing with issues of health and others who mock or mistreat them because of their, size. Some people who have a particular religious belief have to cope with discrimination and prejudice simply because of their faith, young male has two ways that he can respond to unfavorable conditions. He can choose to complain and become a victim of a situation or he can choose to use the situation to motivate himself to overcome obstacles. Blaming Caucasians, foreigners, women or others for his present condition after counterproductive. Blaming others does not serve any reasonable purpose because it wastes energy that could be used to become successful. recognize that any negative influence from other, people are temporary he has the power, he needs to overcome negative people and events in his life all he has to do is choose to use this power to his advantage. Let people who create obstacles for, him serve as a motivating influence.

EXERCISE 3.6 (CONT.)

A young man's energy is a precious commodity. The energy he puts into complaining and blaming others is energy that he could use to move forward as a leader, in life. The greatest challenge that he has is getting a clear vision of the successful male leader that he wants to become.

The next step is to establish important goals with specific dates for accomplishing them. For example, a young man might want to own a home building business with a goal of building 100 homes per year, beginning 10 years from today. (Remember to write into the goals the exact month, day, and year for accomplishing these goals.)

The he decides what it will take for him to achieve the goal he monitors his progress toward the attainment of skills or resources to achieve the goal. He does not wait for anyone else to check his success as he works toward his goals. He checks himself weekly and writes down how far. He has progressed toward his targets.

THIS IS AN IMPORTANT PART OF BEING A MAN WHO IS SERIOUS ABOUT BECOMING SUCCESSFUL.

USE RESILIENCY NETWORKING TO WEAVE TOGETHER A HEALTHIER PLACE TO LIVE FOR EVERYONE. THIS IS AN IMPORTANT PART OF BEING AN AUTHENTIC MAN. THIS IS A GENUINE LEADER.

EXERCISE 3.6(CONT.)
MANHOOD SUCCESS PLAN

Name_____

Complete your plan for success in life by following the example below. List each item in details

SITUATIONS FOR GOAL SETTING	ACTIONS TO BE TAKEN	MEASURABLE SUCCESS MARKER	TIMELINE
Example 1, In my school	I will completely fill out	Two application for computer training program in building construction	By June 1 of a selected year (Example 2050)
Example 2, In my community	I will open a home building business	With five employees	By June 1 of a selected year (Example 2050
1. in my personal life,	I will		By (date) _____ of _____ year.
2. in my house,	I will		By (date) _____ of _____ year.
3. In my family,	I will		By (date) _____ of _____ year.
4. In my school,	I will		By (date) _____ of _____ year.
5. With my friends	I will		By (date) _____ of _____ year.
6. In my community	I will		By (date) _____ of _____ year.
7. In 5 years	I will		

TURNING BOYS INTO MEN A MULTICULTURAL BEHAVIORAL APPROACH

HEALTH AND FITNESS

LESSON 4

TURNING BOYS INTO MEN II
A MULTICULTURAL BEHAVIORAL APPROACH
HEALTH AND FITNESS
LESSON 4

LEARNING OBJECTIVES

You will learn about:

❖ Healthy eating patterns.

❖ Ways in which exercise helps to maintain optimum health.

❖ Ways in which healthy eating and exercise work hand-in-hand to promote healthy living.

❖ Stress reduction

EXERCISE 4.1
CONDITIONING FOR OPTIMAL HEALTH
BOYHOOD TO MANHOOD

Your health is your wealth

Eat to live, don't just live to eat.

FOUNDATION

Have you ever thought about how important it is to take care of your body? Does eating a balanced meal, maintaining a weight that is age, body type, and height appropriate mean anything to you? Young males must address these questions head head-on. A healthy individual is one who works to improve all aspects of himself. One area of a person's life must not be neglected for the other. Understanding the best ways to become mature inside and outside is important. A well-rounded man makes sure to take care of his body from top to bottom. He nurtures, all parts of who he is must move toward and seeks to be in top condition to maintain ideal health and the best possible level of success in life. The goal for maturing males is to begin to better understand better the importance of taking care of the total you. Young people sometimes experience diseases and healthy conditions just as older people but they can stop many health problems in their tracks while they are young by taking excellent care of themselves. This is a core part of being a responsible, mature man.

According to the U.S Centers for Disease Control and Prevention (CDC), overweight is common. For example, 18.5% young people out of 100 are overweighting (obese). This amounts to 13.7 million obese children and adolescents. In 2015-2016, the prevalence of obesity was 39.8% in adults and 18.5% in youth. The prevalence of obesity was higher among middle-aged adults (42.8%) than among younger adults (35.7%). (National Center for Health Statistics, 2017, October, No. 288).

How can you keep this from becoming a problem for you? Good nutrition is necessary in order to provide fuel for the body and nutrients for proper body functioning. Guidelines for healthy eating continue to change as we learn more about good eating practices. The CDC continually updates its recommendations about good eating habits. Current recommendations are listed in a brochure called "Choose Your Plate". Here are some of their recommendations:

Centers for Disease Control & Prevention-Nutritional Recommendations

These recommendations have not changed very much in the last decade. Examples of these dietary recommendations are as follows:

- ❖ Make half your plate fruits and vegetables.
- ❖ Eat red, orange, and dark-green vegetables, such as tomatoes, sweet potatoes, and broccoli, in main and side dishes.
- ❖ Eat fruit, vegetables, or unsalted nuts as snacks - they are nature's original fast foods. Switch to skim or 1% milk. (They have the same amount of calcium and other essential nutrients as whole milk, but less fat and calories.)
- ❖ Try calcium-fortified soy products as an alternative to dairy foods.
- ❖ Make at least half your grains whole.
- ❖ Choose 100% wholegrain cereals, breads, crackers, rice, and pasta.
- ❖ Check the ingredients list on food packages to find whole-grain foods. Vary your protein food choices.

❖ Twice a week, make seafood the protein on your plate.

❖ Eat beans, which are a natural source of fiber and protein.

❖ Keep meat and poultry portions small and lean. Keep your food safe to eat. Learn more at: www.FoodSafety.gov.

A well-rounded teen has the responsibility of keeping up with these changing recommendations as he grows into manhood and beyond this transition. Young males need to take in only the number of calories that experts say is healthy. Overeating is unhealthy, just like under-eating. Record how much food you eat daily and stay within that amount.

Scientific studies prove that eating the right amount of food may help you to live longer. Young men have to be careful in this way to live a long, high high-quality life.

FOOD FOR THOUGHT

1. How well do these guidelines fit with the way that you lead your life?

2. What would you need to do to change the way that you live in order to comply with these guidelines?

3. How willing are you to eat like this?

4. What does good nutrition and exercise have to do with being a well-rounded man?

EXERCISE 4.2
STRESS MANAGEMENT AND ITS EFFECT ON MANHOOD
WHAT DO YOU THINK ABOUT WAYS TO HANDLE STRESS IN YOUR LIFE?

Most often, we think of health in terms of our physical health only, but mental health is just as important. One area of mental health that young men are concerned with is stress. Stress plagues many people. How do we effectively deal with the discomfort of the pressures of life? How do we cope with this uneasiness that is often associated with stress? How do healthy young people deal with societal stressors that affect people, especially male youth?

It is important to identify the source of discomfort. This usually happens through a problem-solving process or a process of elimination of less desirable life choices. Although it is not always possible to determine why a young man feels the way he does, one effective way to handle stress is through exercise.

Exercise helps to relieve tension and promote relaxation after a hard workout. It is vital to maintain a bodyweight that is appropriate for your physical size, height, and bone structure. It is easier to bum calories and reduce stress when you are fit. You can move a trim and lean body more smoothly.

A life with less stress can help keep your blood pressure lower, and you are likely to eat less food unnecessarily. This enables you to be less prone to heart attacks and strokes ("brain attacks") as you get older. Sometimes a young man who deviates from a healthy nutrition plan uses food as a comforter. Talking to a counselor, parents, or a responsible and trustworthy confidant can be an effective

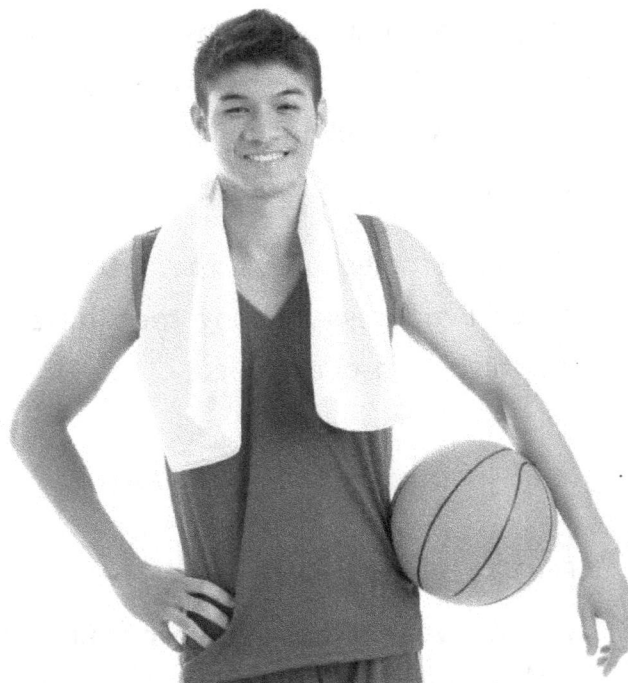

way to keep stress at a level that is low enough so that eating to offset stress is far less necessary.

Young people are as vulnerable to unintended injuries as other age groups. Therefore, it makes sense to be prepared if an unexpected injury occurs. Remember that being in peak mental and physical condition can help you recover from unintentional injuries like car accidents, sports injuries, falls, or other unhealthy events.

Discussion questions

1. What is a "brain attack?"
2. How is a "brain attack" like a heart attack?
3. How well-equipped do you think you are to handle stress in your life?
4. What measures do you think you will need to take to respond to stress in life as you get older?
5. What are the most important sources of stress in your life?
6. How can you prevent the most important stressors in your life from interfering with the way that you live?
7. What does managing stress have to do with becoming a mature, well-rounded man?

EXERCISE 4.3

The Body, Food, and Fuel: Comparison to a Luxury Car

Think about a car as a model for ways that your body uses food or fuel. Understanding how to consume and bum the right food in your body is as important as maintaining the right gas and oil in a car. The car has a metal frame that houses all of its parts, and so does our body have a physical frame. It is important that all the parts of your bodywork well together, just as the parts of the car do when they are well maintained. The car requires a tune-up, oil change, air filter, gas filter, and air in the tires periodically.

Likewise, your body needs food, water, rest, vitamins, and exercise to run smoothly. The body functions better when the heart can pump blood throughout the body with ease. Just as the car's fuel pump sends a flow of gasoline to the engine to bum in order to make it run, the heart must pump fuel easily. The car stores fuel in the gas tank while humans store our energy source in our digestive system initially.

When additional energy is needed, the car pulls from its gasoline reserves to keep it moving. The body draws its energy from the food taken in daily. When the energy level falls short, the fuel reserve in which the fat cells store is used to keep the body going. The engine is the heart of the car, and it has to run smoothly or the rest of the car will not function properly. The same applies to the heart. It cannot beat and pump blood effectively if it is clogged with cholesterol and plaque deposits.

The tires on the car represent the arms and legs of the human. The tires are needed for movement. The legs and arms are used for the movement of our bodies. The tires must remain inflated properly, and the muscles must be toned and in good working order for a young man like you to walk, grasp objects, and carry items efficiently.

The body is perfectly made and requires that a young leader give it the best attention he can to be healthy in all areas. Mental health requires a healthy body to function the way it is intended. We do not think very well if we have had too little sleep, for example. Loving ourselves enough to take care of our mental health is a very important step for a person to take to lead friends, family, and the community in a positive direction.

Discussion questions

1. Which parts of this comparison of a car to the way your body works makes the most sense to you? Explain why.
2. What is your responsibility as a man for seeing to it that all aspects of elements that affect your health fit well together?
3. How can you work with your family and friends to keep you in line with these recommendations for nutrition, exercise, and stress management?
4. What are some ways that you can use computer applications and devices to keep a record of your health habits?
5. How can you use this information to reach health goals?

EXERCISE 4.4

This form is as an example of a food intake recording tool. Read it carefully. Consider using electronic methods to save this information.

TABLE 1 THE HEALTHY MAN A DAY'S FOOD INTAKE RECORD
Write down what you eat and how much, Breakfast I ate the following foods: 1. _____ 2. _____ 3. _____ 4. _____ 5. _____
Write down what you eat and how much, Breakfast I ate the following foods: 1. _____ 2. _____ 3. _____ 4. _____ 5. _____
Write down what you eat and how much, Snacks I ate the following foods: 1. _____ 2. _____ 3. _____ 4. _____ 5. _____
Write down what you eat and how much, Lunch I ate the following foods: 1. _____ 2. _____ 3. _____ 4. _____ 5. _____
Write down what you eat and how much, Snacks I ate the following foods: 1. _____ 2. _____ 3. _____ 4. _____ 5. _____
Write down what you eat and how much, Dinner I ate the following foods: _____ 2. _____ 3. _____ 4. _____ 5. _____
Write down what you eat and how much, Snack before bedtime I ate the following foods: _____ 2. _____ 3. _____ 4. _____ 5. _____

EXERCISE 4.4
YOUR BODY: HOW FIT ARE YOU?
STEPS: WHAT YOU DO
The group leader will give you directions for the following class activities.

Mini-fitness Course
(Make sure that your doctor says that it is fine acceptable for you to perform this exercise before you do it.) Set up an exercise space in a room. Do exercises like basic muscle toning, aerobics, and flexibility. Describe what body responses would tell you that you are in shape or out of shape. What do you think you should do about what you learn from this process?

Healthy Taste Testing Party
Have a taste testing party. Consider making healthy smoothies. (Make sure that no one has any food allergies or conditions that would prevent them from eating specific foods like nuts, vegetables, etc.) Consider making smoothies with fruits and vegetables. Bring in fruits, vegetables, nuts, and other healthy foods for participants to sample. Gather health foods to sample during the party. Take a vote among the group participants to see which health foods and recipes are the most popular winners among the samples for the day.

Stress Reducer
Learn alternatives for reducing stress through problem problem-solving.

Problem Solving Steps
❖ Define what the problem is.
❖ List possible solutions to the problem.
❖ Consider the costs and benefits associated with each solution.
❖ Select a solution.
❖ Put the solution into action
❖ Check to see if the solution really solved the problem.
❖ Start over again if necessary.

Note, however, that the best approach is to prevent life's problems from taking place BEFORE they happen. Many of life's problems have preventive solutions if you find out what the solutions are and use them well.

Role Play
Two Friends' Stress indicators

Role Role-play the following scenario and discuss various problem problem-solving steps.

Mike and Jamal have been friends since kindergarten. Lately, it seems Jamal has been unusually quiet and eats all the time. He is obviously gaining weight in his stomach and other parts of his body. Mike is worried because he has never seen his friend act like this before. Mike decides to ask Jamal if there is a problem, but Jamal acted as if he was offended when confronted. How can Mike help Jamal resolve his eating problem without making Jamal feel bad?

EXERCISE 4.5

Food Consumption: WHAT AM I EATING?

What you do in this exercise;

2. Create a food diary by filling in the blanks on in Table I with the food items that you ate on yesterday.
3. How difficult is it to remember this information?
4. How else can you keep an accurate record with your computer, cell phone, or other handheld devices?
5. What computer programs or "apps" can you use for this purpose?
6. How would you use these computer-based solutions for monitoring your health habits?

TURNING BOYS INTO MEN
A MULTICULTURAL
BEHAVIORAL APPROACH

MALE-FEMALE RELATIONSHIPS

LESSON 5

TURNING BOYS INTO MEN II
A MULTICULTURAL BEHAVIORAL APPROACH
MALE-FEMALE RELATIONSHIPS
LESSON 5

LEARNING OBJECTIVES

You should learn:

- ❖ About the qualities of a perfect woman.
- ❖ About qualities of the type of man that women want.
- ❖ About qualities of an ideal relationship.

EXERCISE 5.1

Identifying the ideal and less than ideal mate

(Provide a 2-3 sentence description.)

EXERCISE 5.2

Let's talk about male-female relationships

My male-female relationship strengths List 3 good personality qualities that you possess.

1.
2.
3.

My male-female relationship growth areas
List 3 less preferred ways of getting along with females that you possess.

1.
2.
3.

EXERCISE 5.3

HEALTHY AND UNHEALTHY INTIMATE (BOYFRIEND-GIRLFRIEND) RELATIONSHIPS

WHAT THINGS ABOUT YOU WOULD A FEMALE FIND HEALTHY IN A RELATIONSHIP?

CONSIDER YOUR PAST CONDUCT IN SOME OF YOUR RELATIONSHIPS AND LIST THREE GOOD BEHAVIORS. (USE OTHER PEOPLE'S RELATIONSHIPS AS EXAMPLES IF NECESSARY.)

What things about you would a female find unhealthy in a relationship?

Consider your past conduct in some of your relationships and list three challenging behaviors that caused problems in your getting along with each other.

1.
2.
3.

EXERCISE 5.4

COMPONENTS OF INTIMATE RELATIONSHIPS
BOYHOOD TO MANHOOD
Healthy Relationships
One + One

How do you measure up on these items that are designed to promote healthy relationships?

_____

_____

_____

_____

- ❖ Neither person in a relationship can control the other person's life. One partner must be willing to let the other person grow and develop to the fullest degree possible.
- ❖ Trust in the relationship is essential. Each partner must be trustworthy and trusting. Consequently, a healthy relationship is one where either person can spend time with male or female friends without their partner worrying about threats to the intimacy of the relationship.
- ❖ Both partners have to be comfortable with the fact that their partner's relationship with friends and family is an acceptable, if not a necessary, way for your partner to be a whole person. Whenever one partner wants to cut the other partner off completely from friends and family, this is a sign that the relationship is not healthy. Maintaining an unhealthy relationship may not be worth the effort for either person.

❖ Physical conflict (e.g., hitting) and mental abuse (e.g., being exceptionally critical and insulting) is a sign that the relationship is in trouble. Males who engage in either behavior may actually be little boys who are trapped in a grown man's body. They can be 30, 40, 50, or 60 years old and still be teenagers as far as their leadership and maturity level is concerned in their relationships.

❖ Always be willing to seek professional help to promote a healthy relationship. This kind of support may occur as the relationship changes over the years. Stay flexible enough to view the process of seeking relationship counseling as strength.

❖ Multiple Simultaneous Relationships Pose Great Emotional and Health Risks

❖ The gold standard for male-female relationships is staying with one mate at a time. Dating other women while you are in a relationship with one person is not a good option. There is nothing cool or manly about running from one woman to the next. Today, having multiple relationships at the same time can pose a great health risk, or possibly be a death sentence because of diseases like HIV/AIDS. Using a condom is safer than unprotected sex. Abstinence, or not having sex at all, is the safest way to protect yourself. Always protect yourself and others from sexual diseases . These diseases can kill. The more sexual partners you have, the more likely it is that you can acquire a disease. Real men are strong and wise enough to remain faithful to one person.

Make a list that tells which of the items just described fits with your lifestyle. Explain how you can fulfill the expectations described in this passage. What challenges to do you see with becoming a man who meets these expectations?

_____

_____

_____

_____

47

EXERCISE 5.5
HEALTHY RELATIONSHIPS HELP PEOPLE GROW

Bragging about the number of females with whom you have had sex is a sign of immaturity. Sexual intercourse should be a private experience between two people. It should not be shared with best friends or acquaintances. Both parties can grow and become better people when one person helps the other person to deal with life's problems. Remember, you may be placing yourself at risk of being handicapped or dying by having close relationships and exchanging body fluids with several females at a time. Aside from the health risks of dating a multitude of partners at the same time, it can lead to other social conflicts, including physical violence. Learning to be a strong and wise man helps to improve your relationship with your mate.

What would you say to other males to teach them about these points? What are the most important items presented in this passage above?

What are the safest relationships, having no sex?

Besides contracting HIV, other health dangers include hepatitis (liver disease) and causing pregnancy through unprotected sex. Unprotected sex can cause death in today's society. The safest sexual behavior is no sex at all that could result in an exchange of body fluids. As a leader, it is important for you to learn how to communicate with your mate. You can make it your business to communicate about issues like abstinence (not having sex) and using condoms to prevent the transmission of body fluids that carry the viruses. Be familiar with the behaviors that can make it more likely for you to catch viruses. Examples include having multiple sex partners and exchanging body fluids by any means during any sex act.

Any time you risk getting someone pregnant, you place your life at risk for dying early of HIV/AIDS and other serious diseases. The most serious problem that males with multiple sex partners face is the fact that they are frequently at greater risk for catching the HIV or sexually transmitted infections (STIs) during unprotected sex compared to many other people who protect themselves. Examples of protecting yourself include being abstinent and using condoms correctly. (Condoms can fail, however, but many experts believe that they are better than using no protection.) You can avoid being the victim of the deadly HIV virus or other STIs by being the smart. Remember anyone, a friend, mate or otherwise, who would expose you to catching the virus is not really your friend. A real friend will never expose you to HIV, STIs, or interfere with your success. Know your friends. A mature male leader avoids dangerous people and hazardous situations.

Write down what you would tell your friends to get them to understand how serious these issues are. How would you get them to protect themselves from these problems?

_____

_____

_____

_____

_____

_____

_____

TURNING BOYS INTO MEN
A MULTICULTURAL
BEHAVIORAL APPROACH

RESPECT FOR WOMEN (PART 1)

LESSON 6

TURNING BOYS INTO MEN II
A MULTICULTURAL BEHAVIORAL APPROACH
RESPECT FOR WOMEN (PART 1)
LESSON 6

WORDS SHOW RESPECT

WHAT HARM ARE YOU CAUSING WITH YOUR WORDS?
MALE-ROLES

Learning Objectives
You should learn:
❖ How to acknowledge women by using positive, respectful, and complimentary statements toward them.
❖ Mutual support between men and women in various relationships: sibling, friendship, coworker, and dating.

EXERCISE 6.1
USING WORDS THAT SHOW FEMALES RESPECT
STEPS: WHAT YOU DO

Use table 6.1 on the next page to identify words that could be considered respectful or disrespectful to females.

EXERCISE 6.2
GAUGING REACTIONS FROM FEMALES ABOUT WORDS FROM MALES
STEPS: WHAT YOU DO:

1. Think about the following questions and be prepared to discuss them with the group.
2. How do females usually respond when you use words from list a toward them?

3. Do the participants who use words from list b toward their mothers also use words from this list toward their girlfriends and other female friends? (A man who disrespects his mother will also disrespect his wife, lover, girlfriend, etc.)
4. Do you feel good when you have used words from list b toward some woman in your life?
5. Does it make you feel more like a man or "macho" to use these words?
6. Is it important to for you to feel macho? Why?

TABLE 6.1

POSITIVE VERBAL COMMENT TOWARDS WOMEN LIST A List 6 words that you can say to show respect in each space below		NEGATIVE VERBAL COMMENT TOWARDS WOMEN LIST A List 6 words that you can say to show disrespectful in each space below	
1.	2.	1.	2.
3.	4.	3.	4.
5.	6.	5.	6.

TURNING BOYS INTO MEN
A MULTICULTURAL
BEHAVIORAL APPROACH

RESPECT FOR WOMEN (PART 2)

LESSON 7

TURNING BOYS INTO MEN II
A MULTICULTURAL BEHAVIORAL APPROACH
RESPECT FOR WOMEN (PART 2)
LESSON 7

LEARNING OBJECTIVE

You should learn:

❖ Four ways to express a greater understanding of how to treat women.

❖ One way to show appreciation for females.

❖ Three ways to protect females.

❖ Two ways to promote a peaceful relationship.

EXERCISE 7.1
DEALING WITH BUDDIES WHO MISTREAT FEMALES SEXUALLY
STEPS: WHAT YOU DO

Read the situation and answer the following question.

Imagine that you are on a camping trip with your buddies. A couple of them decide to raid one of the tents on the other side of the camp ground. Two girls are in the tent. Your friends decide that they are going to hold them captive in the tent until they perform a sex act.

Boyhood to Manhood
Property: Inappropriate Treatment of Females

It is a male leader's responsibility to ensure that females are treated with dignity and respect. Treating females like objects can make it more likely that males will victimize females. Treating females like property can lead some males to physically and sometimes mentally injure females. When you treat a person like you own them, you are more likely to act as if the person has no rights or feelings.

What Right Do You Have to Treat Females Like Sex Objects?

Males who want to be leaders or role models will not treat females like second class citizens. Instead, the male leader has two roles to play. One role is as a protector of females with whom he is in a family relationship - marriage, brother-sister, or father-daughter. The other role is as an opponent of injustice toward women. The male in that role is willing to stand in defense of women, especially when he is with his peers. He speaks out against verbal, physical, sexual, or other types of abuse of females.

Male leaders view females as equal partners with valuable opinions, thoughts, and points of view. Equally important, the male leader encourages equality and avoids treating females like lesser human beings. He recognizes that this actually enriches his own standing as a human being. He is not threatened by strong females but rather welcomes their strength as a complement to his personal qualities. He is willing to stand up for a female's position when she is right and challenges other males in a tactful way when they make insulting remarks about females.

A healthy relationship between a male and a female is usually going to have high and low points. There will be miscommunication from time to time. Neither person in the relationship is always correct. Most importantly, however, each partner is willing to forgive and tries to see the other person's point of view. Neither person holds on to negative memories about the other person's mistakes or shortcomings. A strong male leader is willing to own his mistakes in a relationship.

NOTE

_____

_____

_____

_____

_____

_____

EXERCISE 7.2
<u>SHOWING RESPECT TO FOR MOTHERS</u>

STEPS: What you do the facilitator will select participants to role role-play the following scenario.

You have just walked into the house after being out with your friends. Your mother asks you if you saw the $10 bill that she had left on top of her bedroom dresser. (One participant will act as mother and another as the son). Show a role play where the son is respectful in the way he answers his mother even though he feels wrongly accused without becoming aggressive.

EXERCISE 7.3
LETTER OF APPRECIATION

     Write an appreciation letter here addressed to the females that you care about in your life. Explain why you regard them highly. List the positive actions that they have taken on your behalf, and find a creative way to say thank you to them in your letter. (Use a separate sheet of paper if necessary.)

Dear [Name of a great female in your life]

_____

_____

_____

_____

_____

_____

_____

_____

Your Signature Here_____

EXERCISE 7.4

CHOOSING HOW TO TREAT FEMALES

STEPS: WHAT YOU DO

UNDERMINING THE ROMANTIC RELATIONSHIP

List five things a newly married male can do to under mind his relationship with a female.

1.
2.
3.
4.
5.

Avoiding difficulties in a relationship with females

List five ways a newly married male can avoid having difficulties in a relationship with a female.

1.
2.
3.
4.
5.

EXERCISE 7.5
HOW CAN YOU CHERISH HER?
BOYHOOD TO MANHOOD
DIGNITY:
YOUR RESPONSIBILITY TO FEMALES

It is your responsibility as a male to treat ALL women with respect. This means no name calling, insults, hitting, or violence of any kind, EVER! You have an obligation to keep from calling females profane names or using insulting remarks towards them. Your responsibility as a man is to support women at all times regardless of how much you think they may provoke or mistreat you. YOU ALWAYS HAVE A CHOICE!

It is your responsibility to nurture a positive and healthy relationship with your partner. Whenever you can, anticipate her needs before she has a chance to express them. Under no circumstances is it ever appropriate for you to hit your mate, even if she threatens you. In most cases, hitting your mate is like trying to beat up a child who is much smaller than you. It's an uneven match, and it is inexcusable. When a relationship is so out of control that it becomes violent, it is automatically no longer a genuine and healthy relationship. You should know you are moving toward a physical conflict when you begin to have frequent arguments and verbal conflicts. It is your responsibility to try and talk through it through peacefully or seek professional counseling if you cannot work out misunderstandings.

You have control over your behavior. You can choose to hit or not hit a female. If she starts the mistreatment first with insults or hitting, let her know that this is totally unacceptable! Work out an understanding when you first begin dating that neither of you will mistreat the other person in your relationship no mistreatment by using insulting words or hurtful actions.

SEEK PROFESSIONAL HELP FROM A SCHOOL, COMMUNITY COUNSELOR, OR OTHER QUALIFIED PROFESSIONAL WHEN YOU ARE HAVING A HARD TIME HANDLING THIS KIND OF SITUATION ON YOUR OWN.

You can choose to curse or not curse a female. Decide that nothing a woman can do should make you so angry that you have to try and hurt her. It is all up to you. You MUST exercise self- control at all times in romantic relationships.

TURNING BOYS INTO MEN
A MULTICULTURAL
BEHAVIORAL APPROACH

FATHERHOOD

LESSON 8

TURNING BOYS INTO MEN II
A MULTICULTURAL BEHAVIORAL APPROACH
FATHERHOOD

LESSON 8

LEARNING OBJECTIVES

You should learn:

❖ What it takes to be a father.

❖ What should the father-son relationship look like?

❖ What are the various roles of a father?

EXERCISE 8.1
LEARNING TO BE A FATHER
BOYHOOD TO MANHOOD PASSAGE
FATHERHOOD: MAN'S RESPONSIBILITY

A father is far more than just a biological parent. He is a co-leader with his wife. They both are responsible for their child's full development. When a man fathers a child, he becomes responsible for providing the best care possible throughout his child's developing years. A man shows maturity in meeting the minimum standard of childcare, even if he must sacrifice his own personal needs and wants.

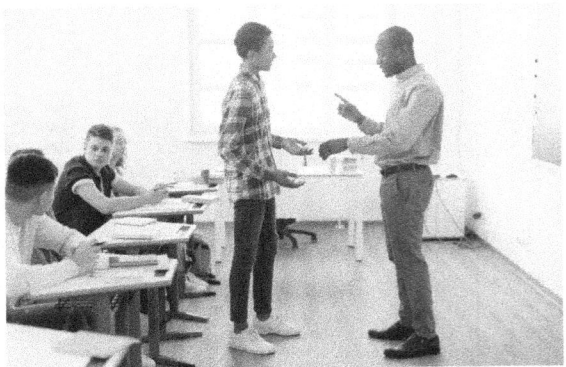

Some males may not have had the privilege of having a caring father who showed them love, affection, and commitment. Some men may be reluctant or simply do not know how to show caring care for their children. In these cases, the father must seek fatherhood training to rise above what he may have missed in his relationship with his father. Real men must be determined to end the cycle of fatherlessness among families by stepping up to the fatherhood challenge.

Fathers focus on the child and sets self-centeredness, criticism, and a lack of ability to be kind and understanding to his family aside. Fathers are consistent in disciplining their children. Fathers must exercise leadership by showing discipline in love, not anger. He must take time to understand each child's unique interests, mannerisms, and gifts. His goal is to promote a whole and well-developed child and a family full of healthy relationships. The mature father spends time with his children and expresses care and love to them through words and actions. Fathers actively look for opportunities to praise the good things their children do while teaching and training where the children need help.

What are some things a father can do to form a close relationship with his child?

_____

_____

_____

List three ways a father can be a role model for his wife and family.

_____

_____

_____

EXERCISE 8.2

THE FATHER'S LESSONS

WHO TRAINS THE CHILD?

ANSWER THE FOLLOWING QUESTIONS BASED ON THE PRECEEDING PASSAGE

How does a boy usually learn what things he has to do to become a man?

Who teaches him these lessons?

Who teaches a boy the most important lessons he needs to know in order to become a well respected man?

What do you need to do to teach a boy to become a man?

EXERCISE 8.3

Father Son ROLE PLAY

STEPS: WHAT YOU DO

Participants will role play the following scenario. Before beginning, the group should suggest 5 key words from the training that the father can use in his discussion with his son.

Scenario: A father is trying to persuade his 16 year old son to change his behavior. The father is very concerned with the direction in which his son's life is heading. The son is disrespectful toward adults at home and school and has been getting into constant fights with his brothers and sister.

Use this role play exercise to demonstrate two different ways for the father in this situation to encourage hits son to be more respectful to people at home.

Repeat this exercise but show the way that the father can tailor what he says to his son to fit what goes on with his son at school between the son and teachers, the principal, the coach, etc.

EXERCISE 8 .4
Father-Son Role Play: LESSON LEARNED
THE FATHER'S LESSON

Answer the following questions based on the preceding passage.
What lessons did the son in the role play learn from the father's discussion?

If you were in the son's situation, how would you apply the father's lessons?

EXERCISE 8.5
THE FATHER'S LEADERSHIP
BOYHOOD TO MANHOOD PASSAGE
Fatherhood Leaders: Many Roles

The role of the father, according to this leadership training, requires that the father look out for the overall well-being of his wife, children, and other immediate family members when needed. The father can serve many roles such as breadwinner, protector, nurturer, and organizer. The father and wife may agree to share some household responsibilities. Fathers can perform roles such as changing diapers, cooking, and cleaning, and that is fine if both parties agree on it. On the other hand, the woman of the house may choose to perform tasks like cutting the grass and washing the car.

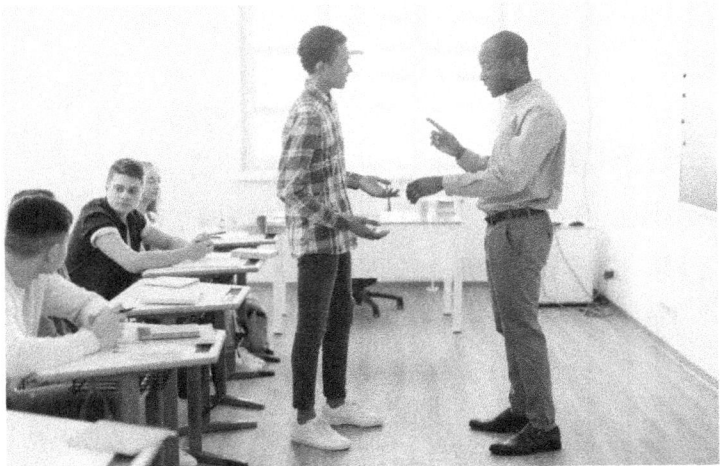

The main point is that in determining the most appropriate roles for the father, the overall needs of the family must take a high priority. Family members must be satisfied with these varied and sometimes non-traditional roles for the family team to run smoothly. Fathers may or may not have the last word in making a decision. If the problem that a family is facing goes beyond the father's knowledge or available time and resources to solve the problem, then he may need to get help from his wife, friend, or a professional. In a family that works well together, the father and wife will be in agreement who performs what role.

All families are not the same. Some are single-parent families. Others are extended families with grandparents, aunts, and uncles, or even friends of the family who act as if they are biological family members. The key is that fathers who are leaders are responsible, unselfish, and dedicated to promoting the growth and success of their families. Fathers are not "friends" in the traditional family. Like a friend, responsible fathers will never lead you to danger or interfere with your success. They keep you safe and promote your success. This is your role as a mature man in the 21st Century.

TURNING BOYS INTO MEN
A MULTICULTURAL
BEHAVIORAL APPROACH

MAN HOOD AND
MASS MEDIA

LESSON 9

TURNING BOYS INTO MEN II
A MULTICULTURAL BEHAVIORAL APPROACH
MANHOOD AND MASS MEDIA
MAKING SENSE OF MUSIC, TELEVISION, VIDEO
AND PRINT MATERIALS

LESSON 9

LEARNING OBJECTIVES

You Should Learn:

❖ About the way that money drives the production of music, T.V. shows, and magazines in the entertainment industry.

❖ About profit-making forces that influence the way young people are presented in the mass media.

❖ Three ways to distinguish between healthy messages in the media versus unhealthy ones.

EXERCISE 9.1
Role Play: Understanding How the Media Works - "Money Bags, Inc."
Boyhood to Manhood
PASSAGE

What does the term mass "Mass Media" mean?

Answer: The term "Mass Media" refers to communication methods that reach large numbers of people to inform or entertain them. Mass media includes television, radio, newspapers, magazines, CDs recordings, and the Internet.

Mass Media and Manhood Your Image and Influence

Mass media can have a powerful affect effect on a young male's self-image and influence because of the quality of what he consumes. This section will help you learn ways to make good judgments about the mass media that you see, hear, and read. You will also learn that the way you respond or the expression of your manhood to the world around you is strongly influenced by mass media. Mass media impacts your self-view. Your self-view determines whether you see yourself positively or negatively. Mass media also influences the way you relate to people in your home, school, and neighborhood. The images that you see on television, hear on the radio, and read in publications can influence the amount of risk that you decide to take with people outside of your day-to-day encounters.

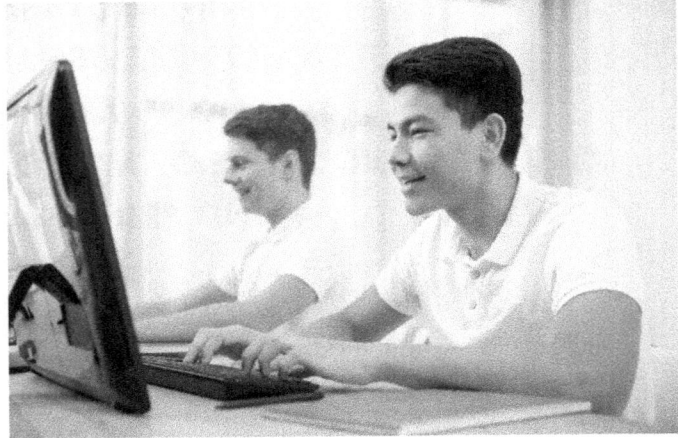

Mass media, or in other words, entertainment products, are created because of a strong motivation for people who create them to earn money to live. There is nothing wrong with creating wholesome entertainment products. The problem is that some entertainment products can be detrimental to your mental and physical well-being. Often the entertainment creator's goal is to make the greatest achievable amount of money possible. This can be acceptable or unacceptable, depending on the way the content of these products affects people's lives. It is the audience's responsibility to decide whether or not to buy it. Never forget that the point of the "Entertainment Business" is to make money for the individuals who create, produce, or package the entertainment. The reason a company usually chooses an idea for an entertainment product is that the project has the potential for yielding large profits. Once that it becomes clear that a type of music, T.V. show, or magazine can generate high sales, the creators may turn out more and more products that are similar to each other.

To what degree do you think this passage is correct?
Why do you agree or disagree?

Influencing the Audience

For the mass media to make money, they must have an audience. For instance, companies recognize that they can draw large audiences to watch movies and listen to songs that have themes about today's ways of life. Company decision-makers recognize that some urban youth can identify with a "thug"," "gangster"," or "street-oriented" lifestyles, and the decision-makers use the young people's attraction to these lifestyles to get the young people to buy their products. Many young people today buy into an urban lifestyle regardless of the fact that even though they have never really been personally exposed to that way of life. In the case of the music, the beat is what often draws young people to the music. It is also important to recognize the fact that many young people like this form of contemporary music, and they enjoy watching movies about glamorous and adventurous lifestyles. Therefore, they go to movies or listen to music that glorifies these lifestyles. In recent years, we have seen a large number of songs that seem to focus on rebellious lifestyles and a substantial number of movies and reality shows that seem to make fighting, drug use, and mistreatment of women acceptable. This did not occur by accident. It is designed to increase the number of paying customers. Again, people who produce these songs and shows do it because it makes money for them.

There is nothing wrong with companies that make money from distributing entertainment products that target young people. Young people must understand, however, that sometimes making money is more important to big companies than the unhealthy messages that their products convey. Some company representatives may make excuses for their products by saying that they are "just entertainment," Regardless of whether they encourage harmful behavior. REMEMBER, IT'S SHOW BUSINESS! Therefore, young people have to learn how to look out for their own interests on the occasions when people in the media try to take advantage of them for money.

CREATE TO MAKE COMPANIES MONEY "SHOW BUSINESS"

Once it becomes clear that a selected type of music, TV. Show, or written form of entertainment can generate high sales, companies and the producers who work on these projects want to make more and more off these products. In this way, they can make more money. Sadly, some people may care more about the money than they care about you!

EXAMINE THE CREATIVE PROCESS

Just about every television show or movie that you see starts out as a book. For a movie, this book is called a script, not too different in purpose from this workbook. The book describes everything that a film producer will need to consider in order to make a movie or television show. Many times, this book, or script, goes through several extensive rewrites before the person who is making the movie is ready to begin making the motion picture, or it is digitally recorded. The writers may change the characters' names, the story ending, or completely change the setting where the movie takes place if they think the change will generate larger audiences and make more money. For example, you can make $100,000 from the sale of one script. This is why reading and writing are so very important essential to making a living in the television and movie industry. People in the television industry need talented people who can read and write very well. They need people who can create an original idea that is interesting enough for people to want to see the product in a theater, on television, or rented online.

Companies want people who can create good, original ideas for songs that will sell large numbers of recordings. The quality of their work has to be appealing enough to sell to young people across the country. Many hours of planning go into making the movies we see and the music we hear on the radio. This is why music producers often carefully focus on the beat in a song because they know this is what young people will purchase.

There is nothing automatically wrong with rap music by itself. There is nothing wrong with television shows and movies about criminal lifestyles, for example, by themselves. Remember that anyone who creates music, books, newspapers, and other forms of entertainment do so in order to make money. The question is, "Does the artist look out for the health, safety, and success of his or her audience when making music, videos, computer games, books, and magazines?" The quality of the content of some artist's work shows they care a lot about their fans. In other cases, the artist's content has little redeeming value in their work that contributes to the fan's health or success. When the artist does not appear to care about what happens to the fans, the fan himself must be responsible for himself. Many personal and social problems may occur for young people when the artist's ONLY concern is putting together creative works that sell. Many people believe that placing curse words, violence, and criminal activity in music, television, and music videos can have a harmful effect on young people. It has been said that it can make young people numb to other people's misery.

Is the Artist a Friend to their Fans?

Young people looking for mass media products or entertainment should apply the definition for what makes a friend. Remember, a friend is someone who will never lead you into danger or interfere with your success. Similarly, if an actor, singer, musician, writer, or company spokesperson attempts to sell you unhealthy ideas and images, "THEY ARE NOT YOUR FRIEND!" It is important to be able to tell the difference between healthy and degrading entertainment. It is equally critical that you allow only healthy entertainment to enter your mind as it is to allow only wholesome food to enter your body. Do you want to consume rotten entertainment any more than you want to eat foul, decayed food? WHAT DO YOU THINK?

❖ Most visual art forms like plays, movies, or other television shows begin as a book, or script.

❖ Good writing and reading skills are essential for telling a story through music, videos, movies, or television shows.

Ask yourself, "Is the music artist, movie actor, music video maker, or recording company your friend?" Remember, a friend is someone who will never lead you to danger or interfere with your success!

EXERCISE 9.2

Role Play: Understanding How the Media Works - "Money Bags Productions, Inc."

STEPS: What you do

Situation One: Have the participants' role play the following scenario. Encourage them to find a solution that protects the young people who will be buying this product.

Several people are sitting around a conference table creating new music video aimed at entertaining young people in the 13- to 15-year-old age group. Mr. Bob Yougotta Ripemoff, the President of the company, is instructing his creative team to be sure the music video has the "right stuff' to generate at least $175,000 in profits for the company in the first month of its nationwide release.

CAST OF CHARACTERS:

Company President: Mr. Bob Yougotta Ripemoff
Music Artist and Vocalist: Ghetto Blade
Company Marketing Representative: Wanda Wooden-Nickel
Video Producer: Thadeus Thuglife

SCENARIO ONE:

Money Bags Productions, Inc. President Mr. Bob YougottaRipemoff is upset that the company has not made a profit in the last six months. The company has been unable to generate hits from the artists who made it famous. The company recently signed a contract, however, with a young man named Ghetto Blade, a vocalist who has a surprise hit that is very different from Money Bags' style.

Mr. Ripemoff wants his video producer to make a video for Ghetto Blade's song that has cursing (full of the B- word), gang-related activity, and sexual innuendo added to the song's lyrics. He says he could care less about who could catch the HIV virus by being influenced to participate in unsafe, risky sexual behavior. He says, "It's their problem if they die from being so stupid." Mr. Ripemoff has made it very clear that anyone who does not go along with his program will be fired immediately.

Vocalist, Ghetto Blade, is strongly resisting the idea of distributing music that could be harmful to young people. Ghetto Blade wants to create a music video that encourages young people not to drink alcohol, use illegal drugs, or engage in risky sexual behavior. He wants his fans to practice brotherhood and promote harmony among young people.

Company Marketing Representative, Wanda Wooden-Nickel, refers to a study that proves using cursing and female dancers in bikinis in videos will help the playlist to generate $225,000 in the first month of release. She says the 13-15 and 15-17 year-old market alone has enough money and desire to purchase this type of music. Wooden-Nickel says the music has the right urban beat, and with some hardcore rap mixed with Ghetto Blade's vocals, it would skyrocket. Ghetto Blade says he will do everything in his power to keep from making the violent music video containing anything that will degrade young people.

Mr. Ripemoff says he will not stand for any disagreement on the part of any artist. Mr. Ripemoff says he doesn't even need Ghetto Blade in the video.

Video Producer, ThadeusThuglife, is not very happy about the requirements the president is requesting but decides to go along with the president's wishes in order to save his job.

Ghetto Blade realizes he is outnumbered by the three executives in the room, and the staff continues to plan the video. They include unfavorable comments using cursing, drugs, and gang activity in the music video. They decide to do so even though Ghetto Blade wants to take a stand for what he thinks is right. After all, the contract gives them that authority.

EXERCISE 9.3

More Role Play: Understanding How the Media Works - "Money Bags Productions, Inc."

STEPS: What you do Situation Two: Prepare a monologue role play using the following scenario.

In this role play, your job is to teach ways to make good decisions about what kind of music to listen to. This time, Money Bags Productions, Inc. has already released the playlist and music video mentioned in the previous story. The CD is full of foul language, sexual gestures, and violent expressions. The company is conducting special promotions in inner-city entertainment locations. Money Bags Productions Inc. is making a tremendous amount of money from the products. Some young people who listen to the music wanted to purchase it so badly that they made up stories to get money from their parents. There are television reports that the music video's extreme violence is being imitated by young people across the country young people across the country and they are imitating the music video's extreme violence. Several young people died as a result of imitating the stories depicted in the music.

In the role play, persuade your fellow participants to understand that they are being abused by Money Bags Productions, Inc. Make them understand that listening to popular music is generally not a problem. It is a problem, however, to take advantage of young people by presenting harmful images simply to get their money. Include the definition for a friend in your argument against harmful music. (Definition: A friend will never lead you to danger or interfere with your success.) Explain to the participants that they can choose to turn off the music and not buy it as a commitment to their own healthy lifestyle rather than giving in to a temporarily appealing, but harmful fad.

STEPS: What you do
Situation III:

In this role play, Ghetto Blade successfully convinces the company to make a healthy video that young people can purchase.

Four participants will role role-play the Money Bags Productions, Inc. characters Company President
Mr. Bob Yougotta Ripemoff, Musical Artist and Vocalist Ghetto Blade, Company Marketing Representative Wanda Wooden-Nickel, and Video Producer ThadeusThuglife in the Conference Room discussing a workable plan for making $175,000 from the sale of the playlist and music video in the product's first-month release. This time vocalist Ghetto Blade takes control and demands that a positive product be made. He outlines elements that will be appealing to the young people across the country. Each one of the other characters at first remains convinced about their individual beliefs regarding the creation of the music video. In other words, they must strongly state their position on making the negative video. Ghetto Blade, however, has compelling examples of playlists and music videos that have made money with positive elements in them. In the end, because Ghetto Blade stood his ground, even when he could have lost his contract. He wins his position because the company is looking for ways to make profits. Ghetto Blade becomes a billionaire because he stood his ground!

YOU JUDGE THE ENTERTAINMENT PRODUCT!
People, who make these TV, music, videos etc, may not be your friends. They may like making money more than they care about you! Learn to make your own judgments. Do sex, drugs and violence fit with becoming a mature man who is a real leader

TURNING BOYS INTO MEN
A MULTICULTURAL
BEHAVIORAL APPROACH II

HOW TO HANDLE
PEOPLE WHO
TREAT YOU UNFAIRLY

LESSON 10

TURNING BOYS INTO MEN II
A MULTICULTURAL BEHAVIORAL APPROACH
HOW TO HANDLE PEOPLE WHO TREAT YOU UNFAIRLY

LESSON 10

LEARNING OBJECTIVES

You should learn:

❖ Ways to respond to people who make negative judgments about young men simply because they are young males.

❖ New ways to cope with mistreatment caused by racial or ethnic bias.

❖ Healthy way to respond to members of other racial and ethnic groups when the young man interprets their actions as disrespectful.

EXERCISE 10.1

How to Handle People Who Mistreat you

Too often, males must learn to deal with the reality that some people in our society view them with suspicion, fear, and mistrust simply because they are young males. Individuals exhibiting this behavior may be Caucasian, Asian, Latino-Hispanic, or themselves. The common thread tying these individuals together is the fact that they all hold unfavorable opinions of young males. Their reasons may be diverse and personal experiences with a few young males, negative images from mass media, or messages they have picked up from others in society.

It is a sensitive issue for individuals who maintain judgmental beliefs and behaviors toward young males. It is just as sensitive to the young males who are unfairly judged before they have a chance to prove themselves otherwise. People who hold negative attitudes toward young males view them as having identical morals and values. It is especially problematic at the public level and many times in private places in society as young males come face to face with their accusers. These are high-risk interactions for the accusers and young males. For young males, historically, the damage from false accusations to their self-concept or self-image may increase over their lifespan. When the accusations are true, they may often lead to more severe labeling by others in society. A small number of young males may view see these encounters as assaults on their manhood and a possible desire to retaliate. Being the object of stereotyping for too many young males is an unpleasant attack on their basically good character. In an excessive number of cases when this occurs, these events are considered mental assaults that have far-reaching consequences.

Learn to Overcome Stereotyping

Let us examine ways to handle being judged unfairly in public places like school, government offices, stores, restaurants, family conflicts, and so on, no matter who you are. The good news is that you can learn to rise above mistreatment and thrive if you handle each situation in a smart way smartly handling each situation.

Young men can learn to cultivate a mature approach to handling people who treat them unfairly mistreat them. One way is to learn to recognize unfairness and injustice. It is important to recognize real conditions where injustice happens because of who you are. It is essential that you learn to make healthy and effective responses to these situations. This is because handling mistreatment correctly can keep you from being suspended from school, out of jail, and other bad outcomes. At the same time, it is wise to avoid being too sensitive to mistreatment. Sometimes a young male is the object of maltreatment because the other person has not been taught how to treat all people fairly. The mistreatment is not always racially motivated. It is worthwhile to use good judgment in handling these situations regardless of the reason for the mistreatment.

Learning to respond correctly to these situations serves the best interests of the young male. It is your responsibility to overcome desires to become hostile in response to an improper aggressor. Likewise, young males have to learn not to let mistreatment from others get under their skin in a way that contributes to unhealthy stress reactions, high blood pressure, strokes, and heart attacks. These harmful internal reactions can add up over a period of time and take a toll on how long a person lives.

Some young men feel that because of who they are, they do not have access to the same resources that others do to approach life's challenges and succeed. It is critical for young men to learn ways to adapt satisfactorily to feelings of mistreatment. You can learn to become a well-rounded, mature man who responds to mistreatment in a smart way smartly responds to mistreatment, and you come out the winner in the long run. Making this adjustment is essential whenever genuine mistreatment occurs.

Sometimes It Is Just a Misunderstanding

Often young males find themselves in uncomfortable and possibly dangerous circumstances for whatever reason. For one, some do not know how to respond appropriately or are too quick to respond to a situation of possible mistreatment in ways that make the situation worse. Some fail to step back from the situation and examine at it clearly. Failure to keep a cool head can place young men and others at risk. This can occur in involve a public situation, a couple's relationship, or in a family conflict. The situation often resulted from a misunderstanding or unclear communication. For people who are quick to respond with anger, insults, and violence, their aggressive behavior can result in jail time, injury, or death. The next two sets of exercises teach young males alternative ways to cope with actual mistreatment when these harmful actions are based upon the young man's skin color, personality, life choices, or cultural group. In these exercises, you will experiment with making adjustments to specific situations which that they may encounter in their day-to-day interactions with others.

EXERCISE 10.1

Identifying Examples of Mistreatment in Your Life

LIST SOME EFFECTIVE WAYS TO HANDLE SITUATIONS LIKE THIS.

_____

_____

_____

_____

EXERCISE 10.2

Handling people who treat you unfairly

1. How could you become trapped into hiding on to past negative experiences dealing people who do not seem to trust you because of who you are?

2. Why should a young male learn new ways to respond to what other people say about him even if it is not wrong?

3. In the areas listed below, what can a young African male do to be the best person that he can be?

   Communication

   Education

   Relationship

   Public image

4. How would you as a young man explain your culture (music, dress, speech) to a person from another culture who says "I don't get it"?

EXERCISE 10.3

Communicating and Working with People Who May Not Understand Your Culture

STEPS: What You Do

In the following exercises, recognize that a critical part of becoming a mature man in the future will be to understand that the world is getting smaller. This means that it is more and more likely that you will need to work with other people for your benefit and theirs. People from all over the world come in contact and communicate with each other more often because of air travel, videoconferencing, and so on. Events that occur on one side of the globe can have an immediate effect on a location on the other side of the globe. People can learn what happens more quickly and travel to other countries more easily. The ways we were used to relating to each other may not be effective now and in the future. It is important to learn to cooperate with other cultural and ethnic groups for the success you may be seeking. Successful men from all backgrounds must learn to get along well with all types of people, regardless of whether they are Caucasian, Latino-Hispanic, Asian or otherwise. It is critical for young men to young men must find ways to avoid carrying distrust, blame, or ill feelings against any group.

COMMUNICATING WITH OTHER CULTURAL GROUPS OF PEOPLE
Why would you be more likely to succeed if you become better able to communicate with people from other races and cultures? Explain.

WORKING WITH OTHER CULTURAL BACKGROUNDS

What are some steps you could take to work smoothly with people from other races and cultures?

1.

2.

3.

4.

5.

6.

7.

8.

9.

10.

TURNING BOYS INTO MEN
A MULTICULTURAL
BEHAVIORAL APPROACH II

HOW TO DEAL WITH
AUTHORITIES

LESSON 11

TURNING BOYS INTO MEN II
A MULTICULTURAL BEHAVIORAL APPROACH
DEALING WITH AUTHORITIES

LESSON 11

LEARNING OBJECTIVES

You should learn:

❖ To display non-verbal examples of behaviors that allows you to respond appropriately to harassment from law enforcement and other officials.

❖ Learn ways to keep out of trouble with authorities.

EXERCISE 11.1

Read this story.

Your parents sent you to the county courthouse to pick up some business papers. You and your friend, Daniel, have never been there before. When you entered the courthouse, you placed your belongings on a conveyor sending them through the X-ray machine. You both proceeded through the metal detector, and the officer frisked and scanned you with his hand-held detector. You asked the officer, "Where is the clerk's office?" The officer points to the courthouse directory down the hall. The directory shows the Clerk's Office is in Room 508. You and Daniel walk to the elevator and push the up button, which lights up.

While waiting, a young lady walked up. She looked at you, rolled her eyes, and pressed the up button which that was already lit as though you did not know you needed to press the elevator button. The elevator arrived, and the door opened. Looking at the two of you, an older lady inside the elevator said, "Oh, my God!" and moved quickly past you as though she thought you were going to attack her. You and Daniel got on the elevator behind the first lady. You pushed the button for the 5th Floor. She pushed the button for the 9th floor, then looked at the two of you and clutched her purse tightly. Insulted by this series of events, you wanted to say something mean.

After leaving the Clerk's Office, you and Daniel discuss ways you could have responded to the officer's lack of assistance and the two ladies' obvious apparent distrust of the two of you.

PEOPLE WHO FEAR YOU IN ISOLATED PLACES DESCRIBE HOW YOU WOULD HANDLE SITUATIONS ON ELEVATORS OR IN OTHER ISOLATED PLACES WHERE SOME PEOPLE MAY VERBALLY OR PHYSICALLY OBJECT TO YOUR PRESENCE

EXERCISE 11.2

Department Store ENCOUNTER Read this story.

Imagine that you are in a department store. You came to the store to purchase a shirt and tie for a family member's wedding. You walk into the Men's Department and notice a store clerk two isles away who is straightening packages of t-shirts and underwear. You pick up a couple of ties to inspect but cannot decide which of them you like better. You decide to take the two ties to the shirt section. While on your way, you notice that the first clerk has been joined by another clerk has joined the first clerk. It is obvious that both clerks are watching your every move. You begin feeling uncomfortable about the situation.

You decide that you will respond to their behavior. You ask the first clerk if he can help you match the two ties you have selected with a couple of shirts. One of the clerks says tells you he has some shirts that would be perfect matches but says the shirts are probably too expensive for you. You are surprised about what he said.

After choosing the shirt and tie that you think go well together, you quickly move to the men's jewelry display. You look for a pair of cuff links to complement the shirt. The clerk removes the jewelry from the display case for you. You examine the cuff links briefly and decide you will wear the cuff links you already have at home.

As you are telling the jewelry clerk you do not want the cuff links, you see the previous two clerks still observing you. You walk to the clerks with the shirt and tie in hand. You explain that you were planning to make a jewelry purchase and ask why are they are observing you so closely. One of them says, "Do you want this shirt and tie or not? We get a lot of people in this store like you acting as if they intend to buy the whole store, and then the merchandise goes missing in action." You hand over your department store credit card to the clerk. She asks for your identification., punches in the account number, and the register approves your transaction. The clerk checks closely to compare your signature on the credit card with your identification signature.

SOLUTIONS: What are some appropriate ways to deal with this situation?

❖ Ask to speak to the store manager.

❖ Write a letter of concern to the corporate office.

❖ Register your concern with the Better Business Bureau (BBB).

❖ Ask your parents to call to speak to company officials on your behalf.

Always be polite and civil. You can be assertive without being disrespectful.

EXERCISE 11.3

Handling POLICE HARRASSMENT

<u>Read this story.</u>

You were riding down the street in a wealthy part of town. You were on your way home after leaving a co-worker's house. One of your parents is an attorney, and the other is an architect. You were driving a late model nice car. Your coworker, Eric, was giving you some free concert tickets, he could not use because he had a family emergency out of town. You had to pick up the tickets that night because Eric would be leaving town that morning at 6:00 a.m. Returning home through the upscale neighborhood, you noticed a lot of people eating and drinking outside at some street-level, open-air restaurants. Many of the customers at these establishments appeared intoxicated and making gestures to encourage you to join them. You were fascinated with the scene, so you slowed down to see whether they were actually serious. Just as you looked up into your rear-view mirror, you heard a siren and saw the flashing blue lights. It took a minute or so for you

to recognize that this police car was trying to pull you over to the side of the road. You pulled over, and the officer asked whether your automobile insurance was current.

The police officer asked you to show him your driver's license, registration, and proof of insurance. You showed him the license in the see-through compartment of your wallet, and he asked you to take the license out of the plastic compartment of the wallet. You began searching through the glove compartment for your insurance card when the police officer asked you to get out of the car.

"Spread 'em!", he said as he pushed you onto your car and began to search you for weapons or illegal items. You tried to explain that you were headed home after picking up some tickets from a coworker. You asked the officer, "What do you want from me? Do I look like a criminal or something?" With an insulting and harsh tone, the officer responded, saying, "Now that you mention it, you do look like a suspect who robbed the liquor store a few blocks away this morning?" The suspect may have been driving a car like this one. The people at the restaurant were looking at you as if you were a criminal, and you were embarrassed.

Every time you tried to explain yourself, the officer said, "Turn around and shut up." By this time, the officer's partner had run a computer check for a stolen car and any outstanding warrants that you might have. The car was not stolen, and there was no reason to interrupt you from continuing your ride across town. The only hitch was that the officer still wanted to see your proof of insurance and threatened to write you a ticket. You stated that the insurance card was somewhere in the glove compartment. You reminded him that if you did not have insurance, the police computer would have indicated it when his partner ran your license.

After looking around for a few minutes, you found the insurance card and tried to give it to the officer. He snatched it out of your hand and said, "You spoiled, well-off brats are all alike." He looked at it and verified that your insurance was current. He said to you, "Sorry for the delay, but the next time have your insurance card ready, rich boy." You drove off feeling mistreated and disrespected but recognized the situation could have been much worse.

SOLUTIONS: What Should You Do Next? Which of the following are the best options?

- ❖ Get the officer's badge number and name off of his uniform.
- ❖ Call his supervisor to explain your concerns.
- ❖ Follow up in writing with a letter.
- ❖ Send an email to his supervisor and describe what happened in detail. Attach photos and video if you can.
- ❖ Make an appointment with the police community relations department to express your concerns.

Remain respectful to the officer at the time of the incident. Follow his directions, and go on what your business as quickly as possible

Do I look like a Criminal?"

In the space below, answer the questions based on the previous passage.

Did the driver do the right things to prevent a conflict in this situation?

In this way a real man handles an encounter with the police?

How would you have felt if you had been placed in a situation like this?

How does this example constitute harassment?

Why do you think the police would behave in such a manner?

Based on the evidence, does it appear the policeman has anything against the young man?

Explain your answers.

TIPS FOR DEALING WITH POLICE
TAKING SELF-CONTROL

* ❖ Remember that all policemen are not bad regardless of their race or culture.
* ❖ Refer to the officer with respect by calling him or her "officer", "sir", or "ma'am", for examples.   At all costs, avoid cursing at the officer.
* ❖ Be as polite as possible.
* ❖ Say, "Is there anything I can do for you officer?"
* ❖ Show the officer your license, etc.
* ❖ Keep your hands visible.   Follow the officer's directions.
* ❖ Remember that it is better to have hurt feelings that a physical injury or face being jailed unnecessarily.
* ❖ Give him the benefit of the doubt.
* ❖ Assume that the officer is trying to do his job.
* ❖ Think to yourself, "Oh, he's only doing his job. I'll give him what he wants."
* ❖ Always respond to the situation in a legal and civil manner on the next day or a time after you have completely left the situation. Recording the incident at the time may be appropriate as long as your approach is legal. Never curse or use insulting language.
* ❖ NOTE: You can decrease the chance of turning a routine stop into a conflict or perhaps time in jail by being respectful and making good choices. You do not have to act like a coward to be respectful.
* ❖ Many of the honest officers are just trying to do their jobs as well as they can.

Which of the following tips we just discussed for dealing with authorities like the police seem to make the most sense?

Explain why you have this opinion.

_____

_____

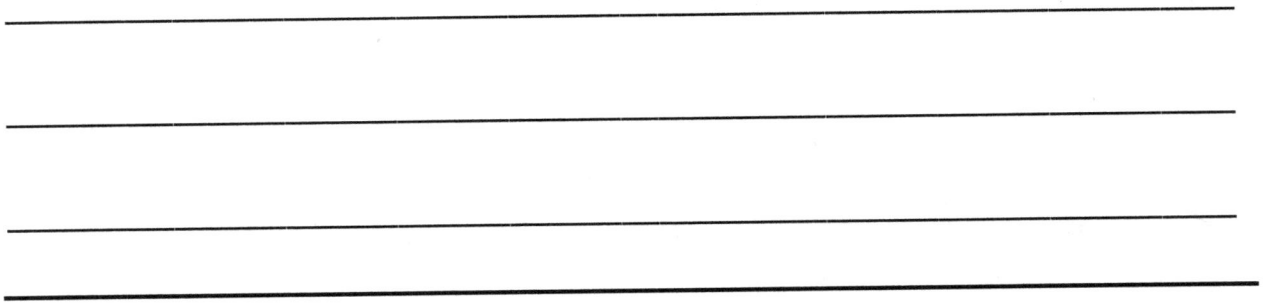

TURNING BOYS INTO MEN
A MULTICULTURAL
BEHAVIORAL APPROACH II

LEARNING TO PREVENT VIOLENCE, MANAGE CONFLICTS AND SELECT REAL FRIENDS

LESSON 12

TURNING BOYS INTO MEN II
A MULTICULTURAL BEHAVIORAL APPROACH
LEARNING TO PREVENT VIOLENCE, MANAGE CONFLICT, AND SELECT REAL FRIENDS

LESSON 12

LEARNING OBJECTIVES

You should learn to:

❖ Discuss ways that conflict affects the way they live.

❖ Give examples of conflict and how it starts between people.

❖ List ways to keep friends and other young people away form from conflict.

❖ Learn two ways to tell whether "a running partner" or associate is really your friend.

EXERCISE 12.1
CONFLICT: STOPPING IT BEFORE IT STARTS AND KEEPING IT FROM HAPPENING

STEPS: What you do Consider what these words mean: Conflict, Prevention, and Management.

❖ What is conflict?

❖ Give an example of a conflict:

(Working definition: A verbal or physical clash or trouble between two or more people.)

❖ What is prevention?

❖ Give an example of prevention:

(Working definition: Keeping an event from occurring before it happens.)

❖ What is management?

❖ Give an example of management

EXERCISE 12.2
TYPES OF CONFLICT

STEPS: What you do
List 5 types of actions or behaviors that show that people are in conflict?
    1.
    2.
    3.
    4.
    5.

EXERCISE 12.3
PREVENTING CONFLICT

STEPS: What you do
List 5 types of conflict that have been in the news lately?
    1.
    2.
    3.
    4.
    5.

List two types of conflict you see at school or in your neighborhood.
    1.
    2.

Which do you see more: conflict with words or physical attacks?

EXERCISE 12.4
WHEN CONFLICT STARTS TO GROW, STOP IT IN ITS TRACKS!

STEPS: What you do Consider the following example of conflict and how it starts between two people.

Johnny (to his friend): "You are an idiot".
George (feeling bad): "Who, me?"
George must now decide what to say or what action to take.

WAYS TO AVOID CONFLICT
Circle Which of the Following Choices You Would Take If You Were George
 ❖ Call Johnny a name
 ❖ Threaten to hurt Johnny.
 ❖ Say, "Oh, he didn't mean it".
 ❖ Hit Johnny
 ❖ Don't pay attention to Johnny.
 ❖ Leave the situation

Explain your choice in the blank spaces:

OTHER WAYS TO AVOID CONFLICT
Here are some examples of how to handle conflict in various situations:

 ❖ Hang around people who do not like to cause conflict.
 ❖ Stay away from places where trouble happens a lot.
 ❖ Protect yourself by ignoring people who say mean things to you.

- ❖ Practice self-control and ways not to let what other people say or do affect you in a bad way.
- ❖ Keep track of your choices in your head.
- ❖ Examine the different actions you could take and choose the safest way to conduct yourself.

BOYHOOD TO MANHOOD

When Friends Criticize

Learn to enjoy alone time

What should you do when friends criticize you? Often people take criticism and choose the wrong relationships because they do not want to be alone. If someone criticizes you, you may want to spend more time with real, long-term friends. Some friends may not be as popular or cool as others, but they may be very good at encouraging you to meet your life goals. When you can't be with good friends, learn to enjoy being alone. Be comfortable spending time alone reading, studying, or working on a computer to invest in your future. Talk with your family about finding creative ways to occupy your time. Use time alone to master skills that you don't have.

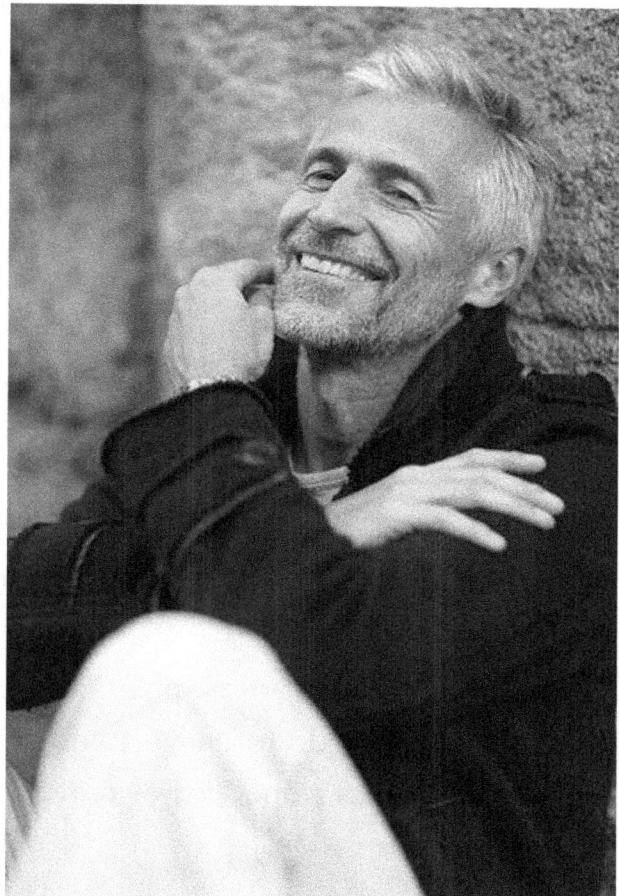

In making new friends, think about whether they are people who you can depend on in an emergency? Would they visit you in the hospital or jail if an emergency occurred? In some close relationships, people want you to be your friends for selfish purposes. They start by making you think that you are cool to get you to think believe you are part of their group. As long as you do what the new friend wants, he remains friendly.

When friends start criticizing you a lot, often, it may be their weapon to try to control you. When you do not know a person's background, you could be asking for trouble by spending time with them. For instance, the person who encourages you to do things that could get you into trouble with the law may not be there to bail you out in a serious situation. This may be because if he goes to jail to visit you, the police officers may lock him in jail for something he has already done wrong. Whenever you get in trouble with the police, many times, the first thing the person does is replace you. He finds someone else who is easy for him to control for his own benefit. This person may be happy to sacrifice your future to advance his own future, to build up his reputation or just to use you for his entertainment. His initial kindness and affection may simply be a way to take advantage of you.

These kinds of friends may be boys in grown men's bodies, as we talked about in Lesson One. At times, although he is an adult in years, the person may be too childlike to see that he is exposing you to danger or interfering with your success. In either case, you may wish to think twice about how important the person's opinion and friendship are to you. REMEMBER: A FRIEND WILLNEVER LEAD YOU TO DANGER OR INTERFERE WITH YOUR SUCCESS!

When conflict occurs, remember that you do not have to let other people define who you are. You do not have to do what they want you to do just because you do not want to be alone. If they criticize, but never encourage, it is a sign to walk away from the relationship.

STEPS: What you do

List three consequences of choosing to stay away from popular friends who often get into trouble - especially when you really like to be around that person?

1.

2.

3.

EXERCISE 12.6

Positive Affirmation GAME FOR YOUNG MEN

STEPS: What you do

- ❖ The facilitator will choose two teams. (The ideal number of players on each team is 3-5 for a total of 6-10 players in the game.)
- ❖ A member of each team takes turns making a statement describing the way he wants to see himself in five years.
- ❖ Each team member must choose a Positive Word to include in his statement from Table 12.A.
- ❖ Make the statement in the most AUDIBLE, BELIEVABLE, AND CONVINCING way possible!
- ❖ Each time a team member completes his turn, his team must show brotherhood by clapping for him. Clap enthusiastically for his positive statement no matter what he says.
- ❖ The facilitator will rate how well the team member delivers his positive affirmation statement and the level of support from his team.

Affirmation Statements-Quality Scores

Needs work = 0 Acceptable = 1

Good delivery = 2

Excellent = 3

Team Support for each other-Brotherhood Scores

Needs work = 0 Acceptable = 1

Good delivery = 2

Excellent = 3

❖ The team with the highest summary score after three rounds wins the affirmation competition.

PREVENTING AND MANAGING CONFLICT
TABLE 12.A
MANHOOD DEVELOPMENT
POSITIVE WORDS

Mature	Fabulous	Decent
Outstanding	Amazing	Strong
Awesome	Fantastic	Incredible
Respectful	Secure	Positive
Exceptional	Brave	Constructive
Spectacular	Excellent	Superb
Thoughtful	Considerate	Marvelous

Fill in the blank with an appropriate word from the above list

1. I'm a _____ young man.

2. I'm a _____ man because I consider

3. Everyone knows that I am a _____ person who knows how to stay out of trouble because I know how to think for myself.

4. I'm a _____ man because I consider other people's feelings to stay out of trouble.

5. Knowing how to prevent conflict makes me a _____ young man.

6. I try to avoid hurting other people in order to stay out of trouble, and this makes me _____

7. I will use _____ to help avoid conflicts with peers.

Affirmation Game
Score Sheet

Team A	Team B
Round 1	
Affirmation Statements—Quality Scores	Affirmation Statements—Quality Scores
Needs work = 0	Needs work = 0
Acceptable = 1	Acceptable = 1
Good delivery = 2	Good delivery = 2
Excellent = 3	Excellent = 3
Judge's rating of the affirmation _____	Judge's rating of the affirmation _____
Team Support for each other—Brotherhood Scores	Team Support for each other—Brotherhood Scores
Needs work = 0	Needs work = 0
Acceptable = 1	Acceptable = 1
Good delivery = 2	Good delivery = 2
Excellent = 3	Excellent = 3
Judge's rating of team support _____	Judge's rating of team support _____
Round 2	
Judge's rating of the affirmation _____	Judge's rating of the affirmation _____
Judge's rating of team support _____	Judge's rating of team support _____
Round 3	
Judge's rating of the affirmation _____	Judge's rating of the affirmation _____
Judge's rating of team support _____	Judge's rating of team support _____
Round 4	
Judge's rating of the affirmation _____	Judge's rating of the affirmation _____
Judge's rating of team support _____	Judge's rating of team support _____
Round 5	
Judge's rating of the affirmation _____	Judge's rating of the affirmation _____
Judge's rating of team support _____	Judge's rating of team support _____

EXERCISE 12.6
Positive and Negative Points of MAKING NONVIOLENT CHOICES
BOYHOOD TO MANHOOD
Preventing Conflict

One way to keep your friends and other young people your age out of verbal and physical conflicts is by staying out of their arguments and fights. In other words, refuse to go along with making the situation worse. Learn to accept other people for who they are. It's OK for people to be different from you. You don't have to try to make others act just like you to feel good about yourself. You can accept other people without accepting all of their actions.

When you master the ability to accept people for who they are, this means that you have become a smarter, stronger, and more mature person. This is how a mature man thinks and acts: Accepting people even though they are different. You can be happy, and at the same time, you do not have to feel that you have to go along with the crowd.

Make a big significant impact in your life by becoming a street-smart young man. There is nothing wrong with being very concerned or possibly afraid under the right conditions. You do not have to get into a conflict just to prove that you are a "man" or a "tough guy".." You do not have to "man up" as they say to prove that you are a "real" man. Remember that you can be a great person regardless of what people say about you. The way to do this is to show that you genuinely care for other people by putting yourself in their places. It all depends on the way that you choose to respond to situations. You can learn how to adjust to situations by performing some of the following actions. You can control your feelings and actions by making smart choices. Learn to be wise by seeking out experienced people with wisdom and character. When you learn to adjust well to bad situations, you become more flexible and more mature.

A Mature Person Knows When to Listen to Someone Else

In scientific work like chemistry, there is a test that tells whether a liquid is harmless or harmful. A liquid can bum you if it is too much like acid or too much like alkaline. When you put a specially treated piece of paper (litmus paper) in a liquid, one type of this paper will turn blue if the liquid is too strong in one direction (alkaline). Another type of paper will turn pink to show whether the liquid is acidic. This is called a litmus test.

Imagine that you are giving a test to the young people around you who call themselves your friends. Some may fail the test because
they are not really your friends. A friend will never lead you to danger or interfere with your success. In order to lead yourself in the correct direction, it is necessary for you to check out every friend to determine whether the person is helpful or harmful to your future. Sometimes they can be harmful to your future without knowing that they are being harmful.

Many times, young men and women get into trouble because they don't take the time to figure out whether a person that they know is exposing them to something dangerous or encouraging them to do something that can be harmful. It is important to know how to perform a human litmus test to judge who is a friend and who is not. In some cases, a so-called friend may try to trick you into doing something unhealthy by making fun of you or implying that they do not want to be your friend. You can be the smart one in the situation by stepping back from the situation and taking a long hard look at who is influencing you in a way that steers you off your course to success.

Choosing violence to solve your problems can interfere with your success. Select friends who are smart enough to work out differences with people in a calm, peaceful manner. This is that the way that a mature man behaves. This is how a mature adult man thinks and acts.

What's Your Test of Friendship?

What if the answer to the friendship litmus test is no, the person is not your friend? The person's opinion or false friendship will not help your educational, mental, social, spiritual, or financial standing in life. It won't help you to pay any bills or fulfill personal obligations now or in the future. The person is trying to get you to do something that you know is wrong, place you in danger, or keep you from being successful. You should strongly consider ignoring the person's opinion. The person's friendship or recognition may not be worth your time or effort in the long run. The person may be immature and undermine your path to a better life. It doesn't matter how they try to criticize you for not doing what they want you to do.

Sometimes the person can destroy your life without intending to do so. On the other hand, if the person is a supportive employer or someone like a mentor who is trying to increase your chances for success, then you probably would want to pay special attention to the person's ideas. The best way to tell whether the person is a friend is to put the person to the friend's litmus test. Ask yourself, "Is this person likely to lead me to danger or interfere with my success?"

One example is interfering with your school work during class time by laughing and talking when the teacher is teaching. Think of each page of your textbook as a hundred-dollar bill that you could earn when you graduate.
Think of your textbook as a $25,000 down payment in gold bars on your $250,000 Lamborghini sports car. Letting a classmate steal opportunity for you to learn during class is like letting the person steal hundred-dollar bills right out of your pocket.

Many times, young men and women get into trouble because they don't take the time to figure out whether a person that they know is exposing them to something dangerous or encouraging them to do something that can be harmful. It is important to know how to perform a human litmus test to judge who is a friend and who is not.

Explain in the space below how you will use the information you learned in this lesson to stay out of conflict and determine which of the people you spend time with are really your friends.

_____

_____

_____

_____

_____

_____

TURNING BOYS INTO MEN A MULTICULTURAL BEHAVIORAL APPROACH II

SPIRITUALITY

LESSON 13

TURNING BOYS INTO MEN II
A MULTICULTURAL BEHAVIORAL APPROACH
SPIRITUALITY

LESSON 13

LEARNING OBJECTIVES

You should learn:

- ❖ How to define two terms: "inner self' and spirituality."
- ❖ How meditation helps you get in line with your inner self.
- ❖ To describe two ways in which the inner self is linked to manhood development.
- ❖ To experience quietness, stillness, and a peaceful state of mind during inner reflection exercises.
- ❖ How to monitor pleasurable bodily sensations during relaxation exercises.

EXERCISE 13.1

Write your definition of spirituality in the section below.

_____

_____

_____

_____

_____

EXERCISE 13.2

Where does your belief fit on the faith and spirituality chart? Explain why your belief fit at the level that you choose.

_____

_____

_____

_____

_____

_____

Different Forms of Faith and a Continuum of Spiritual Belief

Level I	Level II	Level III	Level IV
Faith in oneself based, belief in one's ability, personal experience, and values only. Atheist/Agnostic	Scientific faith based on numbers (data) and testing the world through experimentation Atheist/Agnostic	Combined scientific faith and faith in a higher power underlying the operation of the universe	Faith in a higher power based solely on belief (untested through experimentation and the collection of data) Belief in a higher power as the primary force affecting all things
Spiritual events probably do not exist	Physical measures and data are the gold standard for understanding the world and spiritual occurrences are irrelevant; based on numerical probability and repeated findings through ongoing experimentation	Physical measures and data are the gold standard for understanding the world with the assumption that the spiritual world picks up where science ends; based on numerical probability and repeated findings through ongoing experimentation	Spiritual occurrences are central to everything, and experimentation is unnecessary; Belief that world history and its current operation take place exactly as written in spiritual documents
Belief that what you detect through your five senses accurately represents the real world	Based on theory or a set of assumptions about ways that the universe operates	Based on theory or a set of assumptions about ways that the universe operates with a higher power as the driving force behind everything	Based on beliefs in undetectable forces in the universe based upon physical measurement
Little use of scientific data beyond personal experience	Belief that physical measurements from the world represent the real world accurately	Belief that physical measurements from the world represent the real world accurately and higher power forces are a relevant aspect of living in the world.	Physical measurement of occurrences in the world are not necessarily important compared to the influence of a higher power

EXERCISE 13.3

SPIRITUALITY

THE "INNER SELF"'

Spirituality is a way of getting in touch with the inner person who is deep inside of you. You may refer to this part of yourself as the "inner self." When a person gets in touch with his inner self, he recognizes his feelings and better trusts the feelings that are deep within him.

Spirituality has always been an important part of the many communities. Spirituality is a way of life for many people of different ancestries. Spirituality is most meaningful through personal life experiences and community experiences.

Spirituality can provide a road map for living in a healthy, fulfilling way. Getting in touch with one's inner self can help you to be more in tune with the world. Having a good strong sense of your inner self helps a person to behave in ways that promote good health and wellbeing. Spirituality can lead to better relationships with others. It helps young man develop a good character; -the expression of close-to universally accepted values and attitudes. The inner self also often guides many of the decisions that a mature person makes in order to fully embrace a positive future embrace a positive future fully.

1. How would you describe your inner self?

2. How would you explain the meaning of spirituality or inner self to your friends and family?

3. What does manhood have to do with spirituality?

113

4. What are some of the characteristics of someone who behaves in a "spiritual" manner?

5. What role has spirituality played in the history of different cultures around the world?

SPIRITUALITY IS ROOTED IN THE HUMAN EXPERIENCE

Spirituality is the highest form of wisdom. Spirituality encompasses everything in life and provides a way of looking at life based on a young man's life experiences. Through getting in touch with the inner self, which is an important part of spirituality, a young person develops a greater awareness of his inner self. Spirituality is rooted in the human experience, and it can lead to freedom from influences that keep young men from exercising good conscience, values, and decision decision-making skills.

EXERCISE 13.4
INNER SELF STORIES
STEPS: WHAT YOU DO

Take 5 minutes to role role-play the following scenarios.

Situation A

A young man and his girlfriend were walking outside of the mall after shopping. She felt something in his coat pocket and asked what was it was. The young man told his girlfriend that he stole an expensive bottle of men's cologne while they were in the store. The girl said she was going to tell his older brother who would scold him for stealing the cologne. The young man pushed her away, angrily and shouted, "You are going to do what I say. You're not going to tell my anybody parents anything about my stealing this cologne."

Situation B

You were in a department store, and you noticed that someone had lost a wallet. In the wallet is $150.00 in cash and several credit cards. At first, you thought about taking the money and leaving the wallet and cards, but you decided to turn it into the customer service department. When you telephoned a friend to tell him you turned in the wallet, he called you stupid and said that you should have kept the money.

How could your spiritual beliefs affect the way that you respond in situations A and B?

What is the most mature way to handle each of these situations?

MEDITATION
The facilitator will take you through a meditation process. Afterward, write your responses to the following questions.
❖ How easy or difficult was it to sit still and be quiet?
❖ What about your experience made it easy or difficult to tolerate quiet and stillness?
❖ How were you able to keep your mind from focusing on things other than the facilitator's instructions?
❖ What parts of the meditation exercise led to feelings of discomfort?
❖ How did you avoid any stress that the exercise may have caused?
❖ How relaxed did you feel in order to perform the reflective process?
❖ What aspects of the reflective process helped you to make the most out of the process?

❖ How can learning to be quiet and still help you to develop a greater sense of who you are as a man?

TURNING BOYS INTO MEN
A MULTICULTURAL
BEHAVIORAL APPROACH II

FAST MONEY VERSUS
HONEST MONEY
BECOMING A SUCCESS

LESSON 14

TURNING BOYS INTO MEN II
A MULTICULTURAL BEHAVIORAL APPROACH
FAST MONEY VS. HONEST MONEY BECOMING A SUCCESS

LESSON 14

LEARNING OBJECTIVES

You should learn about:

❖ Benefits and risks of a Fast Money vs. Honest Money Lifestyle.

❖ The relationship between hard work, quality, and success in the future.

❖ Actions that a person can take to become economically successful.

EXERCISE 14.1
HOW TO BE SUCCESSFUL
Requirements for Success

Becoming successful in today's society is not always easy for any man. African American, Caucasian, Asian, Hispanic, and others have to overcome many of the same challenges to become successful in the world. Anyone in any of these groups can become successful through self-development and extremely hard work. Nothing worth having comes easy for many people. Attaining success in the American system has always required preparation, dedication, self-sacrifice, and being willing to stick to a task until it is finished.

In this section, we will examine some of the skills and assets that men can use to earn a good income. Two paths that a person can take in achieving what he thinks is success is earning fast money or earning honest money. Before we proceed, let's see what these terms mean.

Definitions of Fast Money and Honest Money

Fast Money involves earning income, often more quickly than earning making money honestly, by participating in socially unacceptable revenue-generating activities. Here are some examples of Fast Money activities:

❖ Selling illegal drugs on the street
❖ Stealing other people's work for financial gain
❖ Taking people's money by tricking them into making unprofitable investments.

Honest Money involves earning income legally and by providing goods and services and treating people fairly and truthfully. Examples of earning Honest Money are as follows:

❖ Running a plumbing business which is recognized for high high-quality service by the Better Business Bureau
❖ Operating a restaurant that serves great tasting, nutritious food at a reasonable price
❖ Charging customers to make their lawns beautiful in a reasonable amount of time at an economical price

Often these ways of earning income yield large amounts of cash after a while, but some serious risks may be associated with Fast Money choices.

❖ What are the risks associated with earning fast money?
❖ What are the benefits associated with earning honest money?

EXERCISE 14.2

Risks: FAST MONEY

Steps: What you do

List 5 risks that accompany earning fast money?

1.

2.

3.

4.

5.

EXERCISE 14.3

Benefits: HONEST MONEY

STEPS: What you do

List 5 benefits that accompany earning honest money

1.

2.

3.

4.

5.

EXERCISE 14.4
Using Quality to BECOME SUCCESSFUL IN THE FUTURE

People from all over the world come into contact with each other more frequently as the world appears to become smaller and more competitive. Frequently, men who become the most successful are the ones who provide the best possible work, product, or service. Employers, business owners, and consumers demand higher and higher quality. Anyone who does not provide this quality will not be able to compete and earn a good living when compared to men who produce high high-quality goods and services. Therefore, successful men need to completely embrace the following statement to thrive in the next century:

Quality is the single most important item that distinguishes successful from unsuccessful men in the future. The way to success is by engaging in good, long-term planning. That means planning many months or perhaps years ahead. Producing high quality means providing goods and services that meet or exceed standards of excellence. Most industries have standards or benchmarks that tell producers and consumers what products and services are the best. The most competitive men provide high high-quality services and sell the best products. They maintain close, warm relationships with customers so that customers feel good about coming back to the competitive man for additional goods and services. When used over the long term, this approach can make a man rich and successful. It can also be rewarding and make him feel good about the work that he performs.

Your job is to find out what you have to do to produce the highest level of quality for every project that you complete. This is true, no matter what your field of work is. Many jobs have differing, but high, sets of expectations that you have to meet in order for people to consider your work to be of high quality. What you need to do to be successful in the year 2030 and beyond is to develop a reputation for providing high high-quality goods and services. If you do this, many people will want to come back to you over and over before they consider going to anyone else for your goods and services.

In this way, a man gets paid multiple times for a string of great products and services instead of getting paid once for work that is below standard. People do

121

not want to do repeated business with men who perform substandard work. The starting place for training yourself to appreciate and produce high high-quality work is in middle school and continues into high school through college and on the job. What you do in the family, school, community, and in your work life to perfect the quality of your work all leads to building an important foundation for success in the future.

Risks And Benefits Of Different Ways Of Earning A Living

Fast money risks	Honest Money Benefits (e.g., owning your own business)
Likelihood of long term jail sentence	Safety of associating with law-abiding people
Jail time leading to exposure to physical, mental, and sexual abuse	Peace of mind from earning an honorable living
Limited job, contract, teamwork, opportunities, with honest people	Creative freedom
Poor health choices such as contracting sexual diseases because corrupt peer influences	Good healthcare insurance in case of an emergency and the ability to choose your own doctors
Reducing lifetime earning potential	Set your own financial earnings method and goals- no earning limits
Becoming a victim of violence- by being double crossed, criminal conspiracy, etc. (No honor among thieves)	Choice to live in a safe, protected environment
Damaged reputation	Freedom to persue your dreams and passions

Two Earnings Approaches: Fast Money vs. Honest Money

Compare the Fast Money and the Honest charts with each other. What are your thoughts about which of the two is the better choice. Explain in detail why you think one chart is better than the other one. Write your responses below.

_____

_____

_____

_____

Fast Money vs. Honest Money Income Patterns

What do you notice about this person's income level before and after prison on the Fast Money Income chart? Write your comments.

_____

_____

_____

_____

What do you notice about the pattern of increase in income level on the Honest Money Income Chart? Write your comments.

_____

_____

_____

_____

How does the amount of lifetime earnings on the fast money chart compare with earnings on the honest chart?

_____

_____

_____

How many times more money does the honest person may compare to the dishonest person?

_____

_____

_____

How do the average annual income and the average hourly earnings compare with each other for the Fast Money versus Honest Money Income Charts?

_____

_____

_____

What are your conclusions about using the fast money versus the honest money approach to becoming successful?

_____

_____

_____

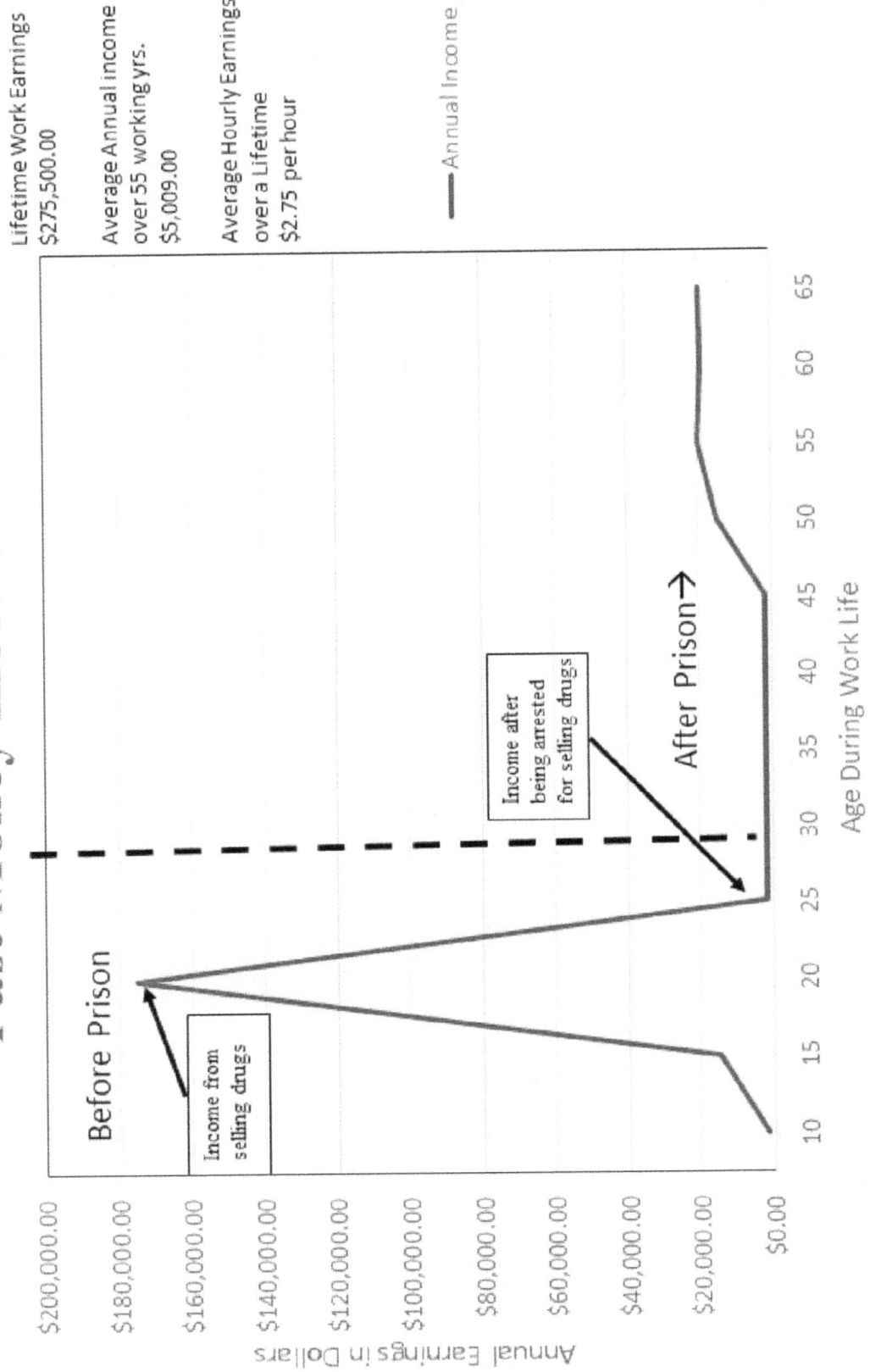

Fast Money Income Chart

Lifetime Work Earnings
$275,500.00

Average Annual income over 55 working yrs.
$5,009.00

Average Hourly Earnings over a Lifetime
$2.75 per hour

—— Annual Income

Before Prison

Income from selling drugs

Income after being arrested for selling drugs

After Prison →

Annual Earnings in Dollars

$200,000.00
$180,000.00
$160,000.00
$140,000.00
$120,000.00
$100,000.00
$80,000.00
$60,000.00
$40,000.00
$20,000.00
$0.00

10   15   20   25   30   35   40   45   50   55   60   65

Age During Work Life

Honest Money Income Chart

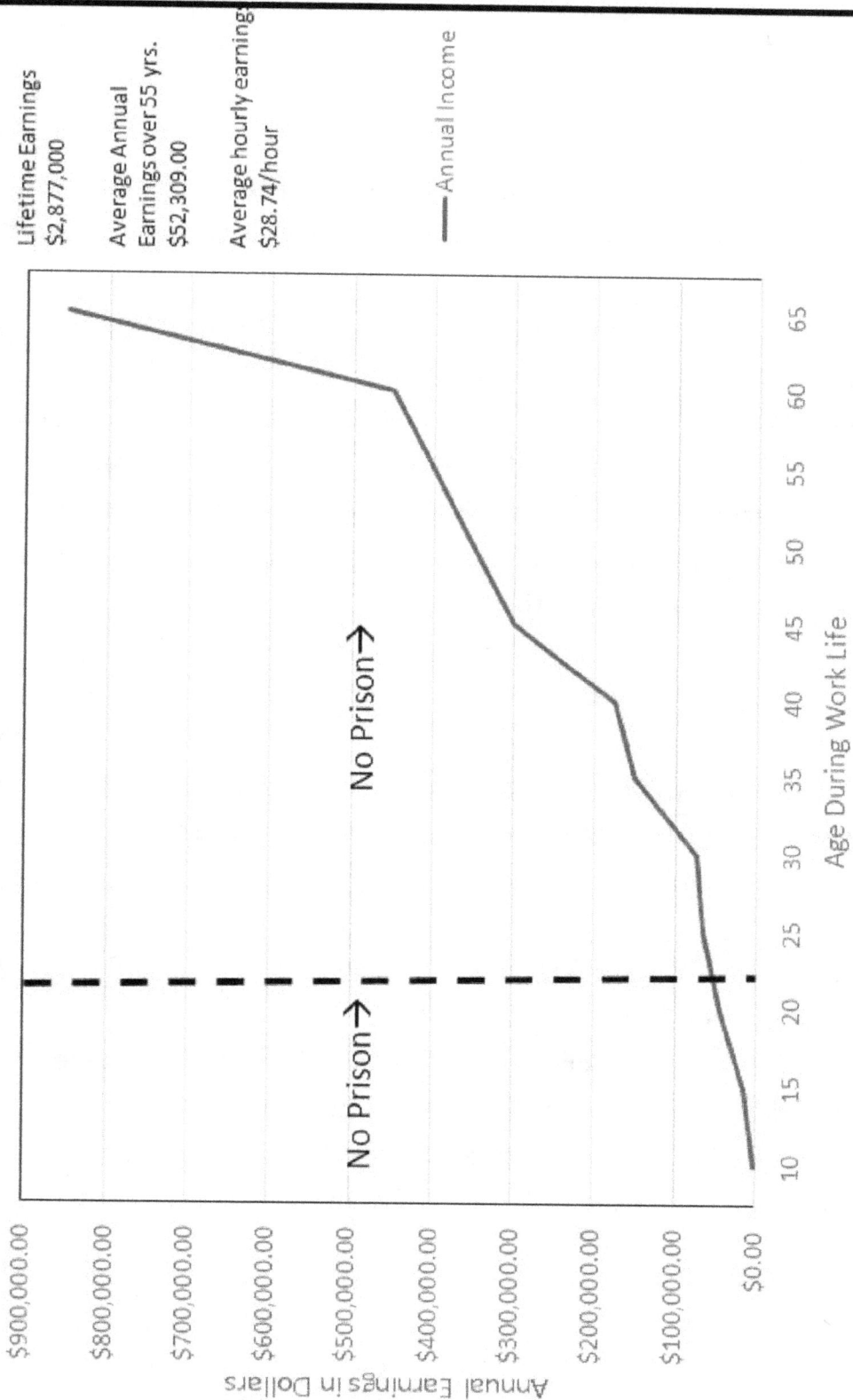

Lifetime Earnings
$2,877,000

Average Annual
Earnings over 55 yrs.
$52,309.00

Average hourly earnings
$28.74/hour

—— Annual Income

No Prison→

No Prison→

Annual Earnings in Dollars

$900,000.00
$800,000.00
$700,000.00
$600,000.00
$500,000.00
$400,000.00
$300,000.00
$200,000.00
$100,000.00
$0.00

10   15   20   25   30   35   40   45   50   55   60   65

Age During Work Life

EXERCISE 14.6

Characteristics of the SUCCESSFUL MAN

The young person:

- ❖ Is honest with himself about his shortcomings and understands that there is always going to be someone who knows more or can do something better than him.

- ❖ Rather than being envious or holding onto ill feelings toward others, he uses others' abilities as a source of encouragement and motivation to do better

- ❖ Takes personal responsibility for overcoming hardships and doesn't waste time and energy blaming other people for his current situation.

- ❖ Avoids waiting for others to tell him what to do to be successful. He reviews his own goals and behavior and makes frequent, appropriate changes that are necessary to achieve these goals.

- ❖ Checks the quality of his own work without being told.

- ❖ Corrects errors and strives to produce the very best work product available.

- ❖ Is realistic about what he can achieve one step at a time and recognizes that large earnings usually come from a gradual movement from one stepping stone to another.

Managing Money: Budgeting
How to Keep Your Money

One of the most important actions that a young man can take after achieving financial stability is to learn ways to manage his money. This is another mark of a leader. He learns how to exercise self-control to use his funds in a way that allows him to maintain a comfortable lifestyle while investing in his future.

THAT USUALLY INVOLVES LEARNING TO LIVE BELOW YOUR INCOME LEVEL! The next step is to plan a successful way to pay important bills and save enough money to prepare for the future. In order to create a good plan for managing his money, the WISE young man must outline all of his expenses versus sources of income. The successful young man's responsibility as a mature leader is to lay out all of the categories of spending and income that he will experience every week, two weeks, or every month. The example listed here is monthly.

It is very important for a young man to stick with the listed items presented in all of his spending areas. The way for him to stick with an intelligent plan for spending is called budgeting. Making a budget is not difficult as long as you identify realistic costs for each expense that you list on the budget and do not exceed your income.

The other key point that he must take into account is to make sure that he includes every cost that applies to him. Examples may include house payment or rent, food, clothing, electric bill, natural gas bill, car payment, telephone, cable or satellite, car insurance, clothing, department store, and personal loans. It is also important to consider the work hours and pay when putting together a budget strategy. Other areas include periodic costs like money for starting a family, going to a trade school, or starting a business. These expenditures call for saving money for an investment in the future.

Some ways to become successful legally are by putting in work hours on a job, a creating and developing business ideas and plans, and saving your money to achieve your goals. It makes sense to develop or revise a success plan every year. Write down your goals and objectives and include realistic deadlines for completing each goal or objective. (Note: Goals are general areas that you want to improve. Objectives are measurable changes in yours performance that anyone else can verify by checking out your achievements.)

KEYS TO MANAGING MY SUCCESS

Think about what the words or phrases below mean to you personally?

1. Self-sacrifice
2. Self-discipline
3. Independent thinking
4. Planning
5. Working a plan
6. Monitoring your progress
7. Seeking out wise people with whom to associate
8. Withstanding rejection from people who say that they are your friends.

Describe various ways in which you will use these terms to achieve success in your life.

Considering the terms just mentioned for managing your life, in what ways to you see your future "SUCCESS" as being financially driven versus your success being dependent on your personal goals?

EXERCISE 14.7

Keeping Control over Your Money
STEPS: What you do

Now let's learn how to keep control of your money by preparing a budget. Now complete the budget on the next page, and then return to the bottom of this page to answer the three questions. Start by writing the monthly income at the top of the chart (For example: $5,000 per month). Fill in each of the items or bills (i.e., Giving, Savings, House/Rent, Utilities, etc.) going down the budget chart page for the following headings:

ITEM OR BILLS, Monthly Total, Payoff Total, How Far Behind

Notice that the headings go from left to right at the top of the chart. Now add the total at the bottom of the page for each of these headings. Answer the following questions.

❖ How much money would you have at the end of the month if you paid all of the bills that you listed in your Monthly Totals'?

❖ How much money would you need to pay off the total for each of these bills? Write in a proposed dollar figure for the total amount of money that you have saved.

❖ Write several sentences to describe how far behind or ahead you would be in meeting the requirements of your monthly budget.

Managing Money with a Basic Budget			
Monthly Income: _____			
ITEM OR BILLS	**Monthly Total**	**Payoff Total**	**How Far Behind**
Giving			
Savings			
House/Rent			
UTILITIES ELECTRICITY WATER GAS PHONE TRASH CABLE FOOD			
TRANSPORTATION CAR PAYMENT GAS & OIL REPAIRS & TIRES CAR INSURANCE			
CLOTHING PERSONAL HEALTH INSURANCE CHILD CARE ENTERTAINMENT			
OTHER MISC.			
Totals→			

TURNING BOYS INTO MEN A MULTICULTURAL BEHAVIORAL APPROACH II

BECOMING A MATURE WELL ROUNDED MAN

LESSON 15

TURNING BOYS INTO MEN
A MULTICULTURAL BEHAVIORAL APPROACH
BECOMING A MATURE, WELL-ROUNDED MAN

LESSON 15

LEARNING OBJECTIVES

You will learn about:

- ❖ What it means to be a complete, mature leader.
- ❖ Little boys in men's bodies—maximizing maturity.
- ❖ Five ways to develop yourself into a complete man from youth to old age.
- ❖ Ways to become a better man and leader by working to improve your community

We started program, Turning Boys into Men, by talking about the difference between actions that boys take compared to behaviors that that mature men perform. Just because you are older does not mean that you are a mature or a well-rounded man. Too many male adults are grown up in years but lack the social maturity that makes them a well-rounded person. Fortunately because of this program you will understand better what it means to be a well-rounded man. You will have opportunities to practice skills and discuss concepts that will help you to achieve greater social maturity and to be a more well-balanced man.

EXERCISE 15.1

Maturity Characteristics

Examine the chart on the next page in order to see the difference between immature boys and mature men. Before you do that, let's look at a definition for social maturity so that it is clearer what the point of this part of the lesson is.

Social maturity: A well-developed ability to behave properly according to social rules and standards at each chronological age in response to people and situations which an individual encounters throughout a lifetime.

The Socially and Emotionally Mature Man

A Little Baby Inside of a Grown Man's Body

Too many men act emotionally like young children on the inside.

Some men who behave this way can have a personality problem called being narcissistic according to clinical psychologists. Just like a little kid, they behave as follows:

- Are unable to put themselves in other people's shoes and see situations the way other people do.
- Fails to follow through on their promises
- Can do no wrong in their words—everyone else is wrong
- Always wants to be in the limelight
- Ashamed of themselves deep down inside
- Dislike themselves deep inside
- Project a FALSE or perfect image of themselves to other people
- Refuse to accept responsibility for their faults
- Pretends that other people always hurt them— "victim complex"
- Takes credit for work they did not do
- Unlikely to help people unless they know they get something out of it
- Prone to temper tantrums or sulking when they don't get their way.
- Get quiet or mad when someone disagrees or criticizes them
- Envious of others or think others are envious of them
- Little or no compassion or feelings for others: EMOTIONALLY DEAF
- Crave praise and attention
- Like to ignore or give people the cold shoulder
- Unpredictably mean and irritable
- Treat other people like things to be used and thrown away
- Little or no sense of right or wrong
- See people and situations in black or white, all or none
- Tell little and big lies whenever it suits their purpose
- Manipulative, critical, and judgemental of others: THEY CAN DISH OUT CRITICISM, BUT THEY CANNOT TAKE IT!
- Pretend to care and love but don't REALLY care about or love people
- Seek one-way relationships only, if possible
- Extremely controlling and have many, many, many rules for others which they feel no need to follow themselves

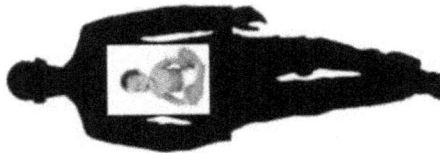

"A small man"

A Healthy Well-Balanced Grown Man

Some men can be 60 years old but act like children on the inside. The emotionally grown up man behaves as follows:

- Other people's feelings, quality of life, and dreams are just as important as those of the mature man.
- Capable of caring and love in intimate relationships with other people
- Hostility and possessiveness have no place in his relationships with others
- Self-love, self-acceptance, and emotionally security allow him to handle frustrating situations without overreacting to small sources of irritation. Easily able to exercise self-control, wait long periods for rewards, and adjust relatively effortlessly to situations beyond his control
- Good reasoning and judgement that is unaffected by emotional distortions of the truth. Able to accept valid feedback from well-meaning, competent individuals.
- UNDERSTANDS HIMSELF IN A WAY THAT SUGGESTS THAT HE HAS ACCURATE AND MEANINGFUL SELF-INSIGHT.
- Able to laugh at himself and use humor in a way that builds relationships with other people. Avoids making fun of other people.
- Belief in a universal view of the world such as a belief in a higher power, God, the connection among universal systems, or universal principles for understanding and living his life.
- Reaches out to people rather than waiting for people to reach out to him; extends a warm, accepting, and tolerant way of dealing with people; active, effective, and strong values which he actually follows for the most part

Gordon Allport as cited in Hall, C.S., and Lindzey, G. Theories of personality. New York: John Wiley & Sons, Inc. 1970.

"A big man"

The Difference between Boys and Socially Mature Men

Choose which column matches the behavior of boys versus mature men. Select one answer for each item.

Items	Boys	Men		Boys	Men
1. Takes responsibility for his actions			18. Is self-centered		
2. Considers other people's feelings routinely			19. Easily influenced by peers		
3. Promotes nonviolence with people who live around him			20. Ruins people and places around him		
4. Gets drunk or high when he feels like it			21. Ruins people and places around him		
5. Earns items he that uses personally			22. Reacts to negative events rather than avoiding them beforehand		
6. Respects people by protecting them			23. Physically mistreats women		
7. Respects property by protecting it			24. Physically mistreats women		
8. Obeys the law			25. Thinks of self more often than others		
9. Promotes people's healthy thoughts and actions among people			26. Thinks of self more often than others		
10. Shows self-control			27. Accepts harmful ideas without considering their effects on others		
11. Maintains self-discipline			28. Starts verbal or physical fights		
12. Makes people around him feel stronger			29. Uses belongings of others without permission		
13. Shows patience			30. Takes advantage of women's belongings		
14. Completes tasks without quitting			31. Shares little of his time or talent with the community		
15. Tolerates others			32. Insists that self-restraint is pointless		
16. Gives back to the community			33. Jumps from one project to an other prematurely		
17. Avoids toxic substances like alcohol and drugs			34. Jumps from one project to an other prematurely		

The Manhood Journey

Becoming a man who is a well-developed, balanced, successful, and mature leader is an uphill climb, but it is an achievable goal. It is also a never-ending process because it is always important to strive for bettering yourself.

Increasingly, successful male leaders from every racial, ethnic, educational, and social background are discovering that they can never become satisfied with just getting by. Successful leaders recognize that they must always be looking for ways to improve or reinvent themselves. Anyone who fails to engage in a continuous improvement process will become outdated in the job market and in the business arena.

One reason why men must become comfortable with change has to do with the ongoing changes in the uses of computers and other applications of science. Computers, telecommunications, and the Internet have all put a different face on the lifestyle of every person in the "developed" world. More importantly, major cities and suburban communities encounters new issues because of constant shifts in ethnic and racial living patterns. To adjust to frequent changes, because of technology and social environments, everyone has to look for opportunities to make dramatic improvements in their value to society and for their own advancement.

Smart male leaders of the future will be looking for ways to get an edge over the competition. The way to get an advance over competition is to become a better you. That often result in putting money in your pocket. This can involve taking refresher courses in different subject areas. It can require changing fields of work completely when necessary. For example, the man who worked as a brick layer for 15 years goes back to school to learn computer landscaping. In another case, the young man who worked in a fast food restaurant returns to school to learn a skilled trade like becoming a chef, caterer or an event coordinator. A man who has repaired computers for five years may desire to start his own business that specializes in making computer upgrades. These men increase their success in part because of their willingness to keep in touch with changes in the job market. Another asset is each man's ability to roll with the punches. Rather than complain about having few opportunities, these leaders create their own opportunities.

They learn new skills, keep up with new opportunities, and take advantage of these opportunities.

Keeping in touch with career opportunities and responding to them is an important matter for a young aspiring male to think about. Yet, earning a comfortable living is not the only area that a young male needs to take into account. Let's take a look at some of the ways in which a young male can move beyond simply earning a living to becoming a well-rounded, polished, and Sophisticated individual.

EXERCISE 15.2
Self-Inventory

MANHOOD DEVELOPMENT CLASS THROUGH EXPOSURE TO MANY ELEMENTS OF LIFE					
First examine the pie chart on the next page. Then come back to this page and check the box to the right that best describes your behavior for each one of the behaviors described below. Choose one box for each item that best describes the way that you act.					
Items	Not at all like me	Slightly like me	Somewhat like me	Like me	Exactly like me
1. I am a person who educates myself by participating in activities like reading, taking formal classes, and volunteering to help others					
2. I am a person who travels away from home (national or international).					
3. I am a person who mingles with people of different backgrounds, education, and cultures.					
4. I am a person who pursues wisdom from seasoned and experienced people.					
5. I am a person who attends artistic, cultural, and educational events.					

Describe your reasons for each of the above five items why you did NOT describe the item as being "Not at all like" you. What would have made you choose that the item was "Exactly like "you?

_____

_____

_____

_____

_____

MANHOOD DEVELOPMENT PROGRAM CLASS THROUGH EXPOSURE TO MANY ELEMENTS OF LIFE

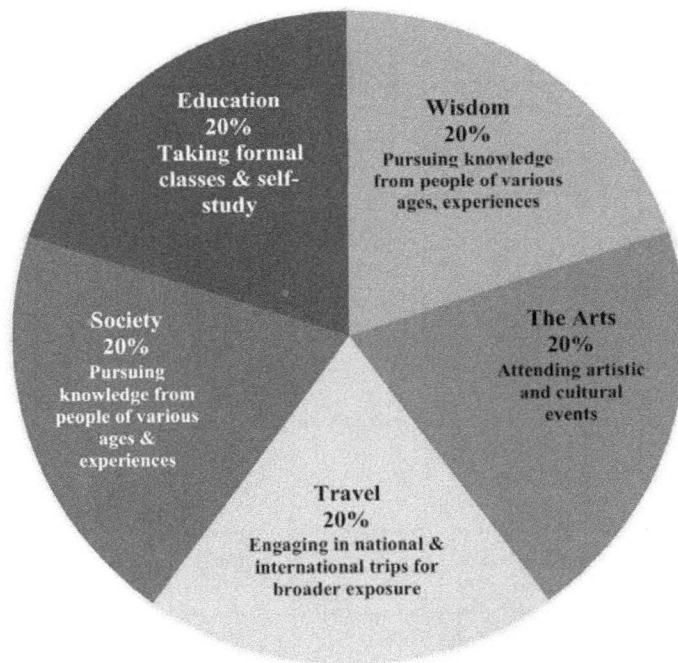

Education
20%
Taking formal classes & self-study

Wisdom
20%
Pursuing knowledge from people of various ages, experiences

Society
20%
Pursuing knowledge from people of various ages & experiences

The Arts
20%
Attending artistic and cultural events

Travel
20%
Engaging in national & international trips for broader exposure

EXERCISE 15.3
RESTRUCTURING YOUR THOUGHTS
Johnny Success

Ways to Think about Beating Your Competition

Here is another way to achieve high standards of success in your life. Image that you are in a race for life against one of the best competitors that you will ever meet. This ideal competitor is another version of you, and this ideal version of yourself is named "Johnny Success". Both you and Johnny have a identical race cars, and our goal is to drive the super highway of life to the top of Challenge Mountain and over the top of the mountain into Success Valley.

This is what you have to think about. Johnny Success is a winner because he is a fierce competitor. In other words, he is always looking for ways to get an advantage over you in this race. In other words, Johnny is bent on doing anything and everything that he can legally do to win the race against you. Johnny is looking for ways to improve himself, his car, the way that he drives his car, or anything else that he can do to insure that he is going to beat you in the race. That means dressing with the latest race course uniform, tuning up his car, using the best gasoline, oil, tires, transmission fluid, brakes, and so on possible to win the race against you.

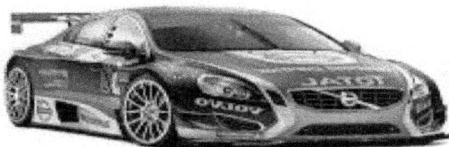

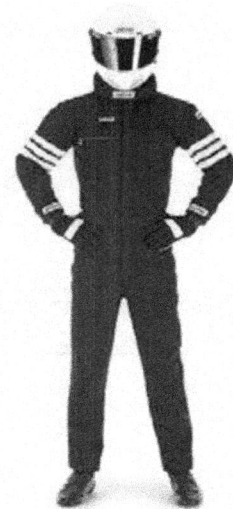

He is fired up about winning at all times. He goes to sleep thinking about winning the race and goes to sleep thinking about ways to beat you. He thinks about what lane to drive in to be able to pass you on the road of life. How fast does he need to drive in light of the distance of the life course so that he does not run out of gas. He is determined to beat you across the finish line.

Now remember that there are many Johnny Successes in the world who are always investing in themselves at all times to be the best race driver that they can be. While Johnny is speeding down the race course at over 150 miles per hour, too many young men are sitting on the side of the road in park or creeping along the highway in low gear at 30 miles per hour. Instead of asking themselves what they can do to improve their vehicle of life, they point fingers at the other drivers. The most successful men strive to get their life in order by watching Johnny Success and doing what he does to place themselves in a position to be able to compete in the race. The question is are you placing yourself in a competitive position with Johnny Success, or are your sitting on the side of the road in park?

What actions do you need to take in your life to make yourself competitive with Johnny Success?

_____

_____

_____

A friend will never lead you to danger or interfere with your success. How would Johnny insure that he has people in his life who help hint to insure that we win the race to Success Valley?

_____

_____

_____

Johnny Success learns the rules of the race better than any of the other drivers so that he knows how to drive his vehicle straight into Success Valley. That includes looking the part of a winning race car driver and outstanding competitor. Looking and acting the part of a winner is called impression management. How do you need to change you appearance in a way that maximizes you competiveness in the race of life? What about your means of managing the way you come across to people could help you to outperform Johnny?

_____

_____

_____

EXERCISE 15.4

Impression Management: Ways to Maximize Your Marketability and Competitiveness in the Business and Work World

THE WAY YOU "CARRY" YOURSELF ADDS TO YOUR BOTTOM LINE!

Define the terms below using your own words.

1. Class- Professional Look

2. Dignity- Noble character, manner or Language; worthy of respect

3. Style-Individual expression of taste in actions and choices

Explain how managing the way that you present yourself to people (impression management) in business and at work can increase the amount of money that you make.

_____

_____

_____

EXERCISE 15.5
ACQUIRING SOCIAL POLISH
Cell Phone Impression Management

Manners that Pay Off with Dollars and Respect

A very important area that has to be a big concern for young men who want to succeed is cell phone use in public and social etiquette and manners. Remember that the use of cell phones in public places like restaurants, movie theaters, professional offices, and so on is considered ill-mannered and undignified. Carrying on a public conversation about private business is considered rude, crude, uncivilized, and unintelligent. You will need to avoid using cellular telephones in these locations unless it is an absolute emergency. If it is an emergency, leave the area and go to a private location where no one can easily hear your conversation. Always represent yourself in a polished and sophisticated manner. You never know when the next employer, talent scout, or potential business partner is watching. It would be unfortunate to lose money by missing out on your next opportunity. That could be because someone saw you as being so lacking in manners and home training that they did not want to work with you.

Also recognize that the way that you carry yourself reflects on the reputation of your family and as a whole. Conduct yourself in the most dignified and sophisticated manner possible without being artificial or snobbish. Using cellular telephones in private locations for routine conversations is a sign of intelligence and being well-raised. It makes your parents and family look like they did a good job of preparing you to operate in society. It also helps you to be more competitive in job and business settings and can contribute to your finances.

What are your thoughts about using a cell phone in a restaurant to talk loudly to friends and associates when the topic is not an emergency? What if you are disturbing the other customers? How can this affect the way important people respect you or avoid working with you? Write out your responses below.

_____

_____

_____

_____

_____

_____

_____

EXERCISE 15.6

Manners Matter SHOWING SOCIAL MANNERS

CONSIDER HOW THE FOLLOWING COULD POSITIVELY AFFECT YOUR RELATIONSHIPS WIT OTHERS.

- ❖ Mouth closed while chewing
- ❖ No singing while eating
- ❖ One hand in your lap
- ❖ Elbows off the table
- ❖ Napkin in lap
- ❖ Being courteous toward others
- ❖ Opening doors for others
- ❖ Never talking while others are talking
- ❖ Never interrupting adult conversations
- ❖ Saying, "Yes, Sir. No, Sir. Yes, Ma'am. No, Ma'am" to older adults.

SHOWING SOCIAL MANNERS

Consider how the following behaviors could favorably affect your relationships with others. What is your responsibility for insuring that you are practicing good manners consistently?

- ❖ Keep your mouth closed while chewing
- ❖ No singing while eating food
- ❖ One hand in your lap at the dinner table
- ❖ Elbows off the table at a dinner event
- ❖ Place your napkin in lap
- ❖ Always being courteous and considerate toward others
- ❖ Opening doors for others, especially ladies
- ❖ Never interrupting conversations or by talking while others are talking
- ❖ Keeping offensive or hurtful comments to yourself regardless of whether they are true
- ❖ Saying, "Yes, Sir. No, Sir. Yes, Ma'am. No, Ma'am" to older adults.

Which of these behaviors could you work on to become more polished and sophisticated? Write out your response in detail below.

_____

_____

_____

_____

_____

EXERCISE 15.7
WHAT IS A MATURE, REAL MAN?

Think about the working definition of a respectful real man. Write a paragraph about how you can become a real man who shows respect to other people with the proper social conduct.

Working definition:
Areal man: Demonstrates respect for himself, females, peers, family, adults, and community.

_____

_____

_____

_____

_____

_____

_____

_____

_____

_____

_____

_____

_____

_____

EXERCISE 15.8
THINKING INDEPENDENTLY
YOU DECIDE

Look at the words below. Based upon what you learned in this training, check either boyhood or Manhood for where you believe you are right now. (be honest)	Boyhood	Manhood
Profanity		
Independence		
Tolerance		
Resistance to change		
Selfishness		
Consideration towards others		
Anticipation of the needs of others		

EXERCISE 15.9

Manhood Lessons Learned: A Review

More consideration of what it takes to be mature men.

Thinking back over the information that you have reviewed in this program, What do you consider to be the most important for helping you to grow and mature as a man? Write out your thoughts in summary below.

❖ Avoids cursing—especially in public. Not only does cursing in public make you look immature, it makes you look foolish and uncultured.

❖ Think for yourself to do what you know is right.

❖ Tolerance for rejection from friends and acquaintances. Remember: A friend will never lead you to danger or interfere with your success. You can always get new friends who will meet the definition of a real friends.

- Learn to make wise decisions about what information is good for your mental
  health. Manage your responsibilities, bills, fatherhood, work, and education
- Treat females with respect and consideration. Be a protector and not a perpetrator!
- A mature leader learns to balance all of these areas for the good of his intimate partner, family and community. A mature leader spends some of his time putting the community first. He is noble in this regard.
- A mature leader imagines himself in others' shoes often and demonstrates compassion toward others. When necessary, he stands up for others in an appropriate way.
- Unless a young man deliberately cultivates these qualities in himself consistently in his life, he cannot be truly successful as a well-integrated and balanced person.

EXERCISE 15.10

NEGOTIATING GOVERNMENT AND POLITICAL SYSTEMS: Exercising the Power of a Man

Learning how to negotiate systems like government, education, medical, and political systems is an important way to improve the quality of life for ns males and all people. The more you learn in this area, the better able you will be able to improve your life and those around you. Learn how systems work legally and honestly. Take the time to find out how agencies and organizations work where people who make decisions do so successfully. Use their methods to influence politics and decision making when the agencies' methods are respectable and legal. Find out who the decisions-makers are and learns ways to influence their decision-making. You have more power and influence than you recognize.

How would you describe the quality of your skills and abilities in this area?

What actions do you need to take to become proficient in each of these areas?

Describe your aspirations in each this area?

EXERCISE 15.11

BECOMING A MAN AS AN EFFECTIVE AGENT OF CHANGE

Learn to access government systems, community agencies, corporations, etc. at points in the organization where you can make a difference in the way the community runs. If you do not gain satisfaction with the first person that you contact in an organization, continue making contacts until you find a sympathetic decision maker. Look inside an organization and outside at agencies who work directly with the one you are interested in changing. Learn how to change laws and policies that affect your life and the lives of other people favorably. Most important, if you feel really strongly about what you are doing, do not give up under any circumstances.

How would you describe the quality of your skills and abilities in this area?

What actions do you need to take to become proficient in each of these areas?

Describe your aspirations in each this area?

EXERCISE 15.12
NETWORKING AND RESILIENCY NETWORKING

Meet influential and seemingly non-influential people and form positive, genuine working relationships with all of them. Never underestimate the value of anyone! Treat everyone with respect at all times! Healthy relationships with other people make the world function seamlessly! Try to find common ground with other people who may have the same interests that you do. Branch out from these individuals to others who have interests similar to yours. The truly mature man multiplies his effectiveness by strengthening relationships with others. His goal is always to form positive, honest, trustworthy, and genuine relationships with others.

How would you describe the quality of your skills and abilities in this area?

What actions do you need to take to become proficient in each of these areas?

Describe your aspirations in each this area?

Closing Thoughts
BECOMING THE PERFECT MAN

Remember that it would be rare, if not impossible, for any one person to display ALL of the qualities outlined in the lessons presented here for leaders like you to COMPLETELY develop their manhood to absolute maturity. Why expect that? This is a lifelong growth and learning process with forward and backward movement along the way. No one expects you to be perfect! The main point is that you exhibit an overall forward movement in the direction that this program is taking your behavior. HERE ARE SOME IMPORTANT PARTING WORDS:

The key qualities that you should consider pursuing as a fully developed leader include cultivating in yourself:

- ❖ Maturity
- ❖ Responsibility
- ❖ Brotherhood
- ❖ Good physical development—nutrition & exercise Strong mental health
- ❖ Following laws and worldwide standards Honest achievement
- ❖ Pursuit of high quality in all things Respect, especially for women and others
- ❖ Genuine concern for others—reaching back and reaching out
- ❖ A violence-free lifestyle
- ❖ A body free from contaminating substances like illicit drugs
- ❖ Ongoing movement towards becoming a polished, well-mannered man of sophistication.

The growth process never ends. The important point is that you do not necessarily have to display ALL of these qualities immediately or all at once. The journey toward becoming a mature, well-rounded man is as important as the destination or goal.

A mature, whole man will always work to pursue these virtues as a leader who constantly redefines himself for the changing needs his circumstances and the world. Yet he remains an independent thinker. In this way, you, and young men like you, will be better prepared to face the challenges of manhood in the years

2050, 2150, 2250, and beyond. Also, learn to give yourself credit for the progress that you make in these areas. If you follow the recommendations listed
In this program, you will be in a much better position to excel in life.
Best wishes, and thank you for caring about yourself and your future. YOU DESERVE SUCCESS!

Selected sources for key research-based behavioral principles used in the program

Behavior Modification and Cognitive-Behavioral Reading List

Behavior Modification Principles and Procedures, Fifth Edition, Raymond G. Miltenberger, Cengage Learning, 2016

International Handbook of Behavior Modification and Therapy, Alan S. Bellack, Plenum Press, 1982

Behavior Modification: What It Is and How To Do It, Tenth Edition 10th Edition, Garry Martin & Joseph J. Pear, Routledge, 2016

Behavior Principles in Everyday Life (4th Edition) 4th Edition, John D. Baldwin & Janice I. Baldwin, Delmar Cengage Learning, 2010

Applied Behavior Analysis (2nd Edition), John O. Cooper, Timothy E. Heron, and William L. Heward, Pearson Education Limited, 2013